D1027170

Concussion Discussions

A Functional Approach to Recovery
After Brain Injury
Volume 2

Concussion Discussions

A Functional Approach to Recovery
After Brain Injury
Volume 2

1st edition
Compiled by: Amy Zellmer and Dr. Shane Steadman
Published by: Faces of TBI, LLC, Hastings, Minnesota

Concussion Discussions:
A Functional Approach to Recovery After Brain Injury
Volume 2
©Copyright 2022 by Amy Zellmer
All rights reserved.

No part of this book may be reproduced in any form whatsoever, by photography or xerography or by any other means, by broadcast or transmission, by translation into any kind of language, nor by recording electronically or otherwise, without permission in writing from the author, except by a reviewer, who may quote brief passages in critical articles or reviews.

First Edition
ISBN: 978-1-7366320-1-7
LCCN: 2022917580

First Printing October, 2022

Cover design by: Heide Woodworth
Inside design by: FuzionPress
Edited by: Kat Bodrie
Copy editing by: Lynn Garthwaite
Compiled by: Amy Zellmer and Dr. Shane Steadman

Published by: Faces of TBI, LLC, Hastings, Minnesota

Dedicated to my Tribe

Table of Contents

Introduction

By Amy Zellmer

"Wherever the art of medicine is loved, there is also a love of humanity." — Hippocrates

After falling on a patch of black ice in 2014, I had no idea I was about to embark on an incredible journey. Like many of you, I struggled for several years trying to find a provider who would help me — and, at the very least, listen to me.

I asked — no, begged — for help. I kept hearing things like "There's nothing we can do," "You just have to give it more time," "I think you're just depressed," and "I think you may be imagining your symptoms." Those words left me incredibly discouraged and frustrated. I mean, these were professionals who were supposed to know how to help me, yet they had zero answers.

At one point, a neuropsychologist wanted to put me on antidepressants, Ritalin, and sleeping pills after a single meeting with me, stating that I was just depressed and wasn't trying hard enough.

But the truth was I had to try *extra* hard just to manage my day-to-day activities, such as showering and feeding myself. It angered me that this doctor was writing me off after a single session, especially since they didn't know anything else about me or my journey thus far.

Finally, at the one-year mark of my injury, my neurologist told me this was likely the best I was going to get. That wasn't an answer I was willing to accept after having done research on my own. I begged her for any type of therapy she thought could help, and she reluctantly sent me to cranial sacral therapy. This was the first modality that had been ordered for me — in just over a year.

Fortunately, the therapy helped and relieved my brain fog. The physical therapist I worked with was amazing and gave me hope just by validating my symptoms and the way I felt. He was genuinely concerned for me and wanted me to get better, yet after about a dozen treatments, insurance restrictions ended them.

At that point, I decided to take my recovery into my own hands and began writing for *Huffington Post*, sharing my journey and encouraging others to remain hopeful. I also began getting back into yoga, something I hadn't been able to do since my injury. I was determined to gain back some of my mobility and balance.

After struggling for over two and a half years, I discovered functional neurology. My mind was blown that I hadn't heard about this modality, and that none of my doctors had suggested it. This breakthrough was life-changing for me.

My initial exam was two hours long. None of the other providers had spent more than 30 minutes with me. The doctor validated every symptom I explained while other providers had just shrugged them off, telling me they were probably in my head. I did intensive sessions for several weeks and noticed profound results after just a few sessions.

This began my passion for helping others find providers who can truly help them sooner rather than later in their recovery.

After the phenomenal success of *Concussion Discussions*, we knew that a volume two was needed. There are so many incredible doctors around the country who have the training, knowledge, and passion to help brain injury survivors. I felt it was my calling to provide survivors with a resource to connect them with these providers!

As you explore the chapters of this book, I believe you'll be surprised at some of the (unfortunately) best-kept secrets in the brain injury community. You'll learn about different symptoms associated with brain injury (balance, dysautonomia, dizziness, etc.). You'll meet providers who specialize in working with individuals with brain injury and who understand how to help you find relief.

My hope is that you are inspired to seek treatment from any one of them, but most importantly, know you *always* have hope, no matter how long ago your injury occurred.

Chapter 1

Living in Fight or Flight After a Brain Injury

By Dr. Shane Steadman, DC, DACNB, DABCN, CNS

One of the most primitive areas of the brain, the mesencephalon, is responsible for our fight-or-flight response. Our fight-or-flight system, or sympathetic system, is in the midbrain and is an autonomic response to acute stress, trauma, or perceived danger. Within the autonomic system, there is the parasympathetic system (rest and digest) and the sympathetic system (fight, flight, or freeze). There should be appropriate times for each to be active, but for those with brain injuries, the fight-or-flight response may get stuck at high levels, and treatment is needed to return to normal levels.

The Sympathetic System

The sympathetic system is a very essential part of the brain, but usually it's needed only in small increments. We see examples of an increased sympathetic system when watching intense or scary movies. We'll see a character go into a dark alley, downtown, in the middle of the night. Suddenly, the person is aware of their surroundings; they see shadows as water droplets hit the pavement. Then a cat jumps out of nowhere, and we hear the proverbial pin drop. This type of suspense is what makes our fight-or-flight response increase until we eventually jump out of our seats. This should be a temporary response where we feel our heart race, our breathing change, and our hands get clammy. Normally, we are able to recover back to baseline quickly with no adverse effects.

Now, imagine someone living in a state of fight-or-flight every day. In fact, this may describe you. The sympathetic response can easily be turned on, or triggered, but the "off" button is broken. Some describe the feeling as their brain going 100 miles per hour (mph). A person's sympathetic response should be around 45 mph, a nice cruising speed that is easy to manage and ready in case of an emergency. When someone is stressed, their speedometer should naturally go up to 75 mph and then back down. A person who has experienced trauma and other types of post-traumatic stress disorder (PTSD) might sit at 150 mph or higher. Their sympathetic system is primed and ready to go with very little activation.

This state of function is not sustainable for a long period without consequences. Like driving at high speed, the midbrain can seem out of control and difficult to manage. Being in a sympathetic response for long durations of time can have impacts on sleep, hormones, digestion, vision, muscle tone, respiration, and the cardiovascular and other systems. When being in a sympathetic response continuously, small amounts of perceived stress can further perpetuate the response, such as bright lights, crowded rooms, noise from children, close proximity to others, certain types of touch, or even confusion at what was said by another person.

How a Brain Injury Affects the Sympathetic System

There are many circuits in the brain that help to keep a balance between the parasympathetic and sympathetic systems, meaning that our healthy brain modulates and maintains harmony through the rest of the brain and the body. When brain injuries occur, these circuits that create harmony and homeostasis become altered.

For example, when there is damage to the frontal lobe, we can lose our top-down modulation of the midbrain structures, often seen in motor vehicle accidents and sports related concussions. A person can report symptoms of depression, anxiety, difficulty with focus, changes in memory, and motivation, to name a few.

If the injury was sustained due to hitting the back of the head, we could see a change in cerebellar function that causes a lack of bottom-up modulation of our midbrain structures. Symptoms related to the cerebellum can include light sensitivity, sound sensitivity, dizziness, changes in balance, and vision.

Both examples of brain damage can increase the sympathetic response over time but come with other complaints. No two injuries are the same, but all can have an underlying long-term response of being in fight-or-flight mode. The sympathetic response can stay elevated for days, weeks, or even years. It's like having the brakes broken and nothing to stop the fight-or-flight system.

People who struggle with an overactive sympathetic response may have the following complaints:

1. Light, sound, and/or touch sensitivity
2. Migraines and headaches
3. Heightened smell
4. Tinnitus
5. Postural orthostatic tachycardia syndrome (POTS) and dysautonomia
6. High blood pressure
7. Increased heart rate
8. Shallow breathing
9. Cold and clammy hands
10. Racing thoughts
11. Difficulty with reading
12. Difficulty with focusing
13. Inability to go to sleep or stay asleep
14. Aversion to physical proximity to others (i.e. not wanting others in their "bubble")

One of the struggles with an increased sympathetic response is that the amygdala, or limbic system, which is responsible for fear and anxiety, can also become elevated. Now imagine being fearful and anxious most every day. Those who struggle with an increase in fight-or-flight and an elevated amygdala can become anxious about "trivial" things — it might seem trivial to others, but to the person struggling with anxiety, it is not a small thing.

Struggling with this can result in significant insomnia, obsessive-compulsive tendencies, phobias, and other anxiety disorders. When these survival mechanisms increase, a person might become emotional at a family function; noises and visual stimulation may create an anxiety response, and the person needs to leave the room or even the event. Or the person might become stressed and need to double-check their routines — an obsessive-compulsive response — to make sure everything is done. However, this process may cause them to be late for work and hinder normal, everyday activities.

Also, what takes place physiologically can have an impact on the brain. For instance, high anxiety can contribute to food sensitivities and digestive complaints. However, digestive symptoms and food sensitivities can also lead to increased anxiety. The brain plays a role in hormone cycles as well, and at certain times during the cycle, a person can experience an increase in sympathetic responses.

Treatment for an Out-of-Control Sympathetic System

The big question becomes: What can be done to help manage an increased sympathetic response? Or what can be done when it speeds up and goes out of control?

The first step is to identify the causes or triggers and to reduce them as much as possible. Anything that creates a stress response can result in a fight-or-flight response. This can range from a food allergy to a stressful relationship.

Counseling can be an important step in working on relationships, past traumas, and other causes of PTSD. Stress reduction techniques can also help, including relaxation, breathing exercises, and meditation programs. There are many programs that can be downloaded as an app that are inexpensive or free. Also, using equipment like blue-blocking glasses or rose-colored glasses can help reduce light and high-frequency lights that contribute to an increased sympathetic response.

The next step is to work on the metabolic system, which involves balancing hormones, stabilizing blood sugar, and normalizing adrenal function, thyroid function, and even iron levels. Having a deficiency of these components, or any other type of endocrine imbalance, can impact brain function, cause inflammation, and create internal stress, which then leads to a sympathetic response.

Eating healthy, taking walks, and stabilizing blood sugar are just a few of the ways to reduce inflammation. Supplements can also be used, including fish oil, glutathione, turmeric, adrenals, and even neurotransmitters like gamma-aminobutyric acid (GABA).

Finally, working with someone who understands functional neurology can be beneficial. The brain is very integrated and is much like an orchestra where everything should be in sync and harmonized. When certain areas of the brain are out of tune, the sound is not as pleasant as it should be. A functional neurologist understands the brain's proper functioning and is able to diagnose the dysfunction and develop a course of treatment.

The goal in understanding neurophysiology is to make sense of why a person struggles with symptoms such as anxiety, light sensitivity, sound sensitivity, or insomnia after a brain injury. Having an exam that looks at the different areas of the brain is important for developing a treatment plan to help the orchestra sound great again.

Conclusion

After a comprehensive workup, a treatment plan should consist of brain-based therapies and metabolic support, and if needed, diet and supplemental support, along with counseling, neurotransmitter support, and self-care. Unfortunately, there is not a protocol or one-size-fits-all remedy to guide and advocate through the journey of healing.

Managing a stress response often needs a team approach. Counseling, metabolic support, and neurological support can be a winning team. Going through this process of making improvements to reduce the sympathetic system and improve overall brain function may feel like trial and error, but each person is different, with their own history and imbalances. Starting somewhere and celebrating the small victories will help you stick to the right path. It may be long, but there is hope.

Dr. Shane Steadman is owner and clinic director of Integrated Brain Centers in Denver, Colorado. He is a board-certified chiropractic neurologist and a chiropractic nutritionist. He has been lecturing since 2006, speaking to healthcare professionals on the testing and clinical applications of functional endocrinology, immunology, and blood chemistry. Dr. Steadman travels across the country lecturing on topics such as introduction to neurochemistry, applied brain concepts and clinical nutrition, functional endocrinology, migraines, and nutritional management of neurodegenerative diseases. In 2014, Dr. Steadman was awarded Educator of the Year by the International Association of Neurology and Rehabilitation. He has also been interviewed via TV, radio, and podcast concerning various subjects on brain function.

Chapter 2

The Role of Neck Trauma in Brain Injury Symptoms and Recovery
By Dr. Ayla Wolf, DAOM, L.Ac., Dipl. OM (NCCAOM)

Brain injuries often involve simultaneous trauma to the neck. Some of the most common persistent symptoms people experience after a traumatic brain injury (TBI) are dizziness, disequilibrium, headaches, chronic neck tension, blurry vision, and nausea. These symptoms can also occur as a result of a traumatic injury to the neck even in the absence of a brain injury. In this chapter, we will examine the importance of neck trauma and how it drives these debilitating symptoms, as well as how an integrated neurological rehab program can be the solution.

Dizziness, Vertigo, and Disequilibrium: Lack of Sensory Integration

The ability to accurately describe and communicate one's experience allows for better diagnoses when working with providers. Many drivers contribute to dizziness, so a skilled clinician will ask questions about the exact situations that elicit such moments, such as whether the dizziness occurs when changing positions from sitting to standing or from turning the head too fast, or when there is a lot of visual movement taking place.

Teasing out specific triggers is key for an accurate diagnosis. It is also useful to distinguish a sense of dizziness from true vertigo and from disequilibrium, which are different experiences:

1. Dizziness is a sense of disturbed or impaired spatial orientation without a false or distorted sense of motion. When this is a result of neck trauma, it is called cervicogenic dizziness.
2. Vertigo can be a false perception of self-movement when you are at rest and not moving. You may feel that the world is spinning around you or that you are rotating. But it can also be the feeling of distorted self-motion with normal movement, meaning that as you move, you may feel a sense that the movement is much greater than what is actually occurring.
3. Disequilibrium can be described as an inability to maintain physical balance or the feeling of being unstable. This can occur while seated, standing, or walking.

Recognizing the difference between dizziness, vertigo, and disequilibrium is essential for a practitioner in correctly identifying the underlying imbalances and determining the best treatment plan, and it is important to understand why and how neck trauma can cause these debilitating symptoms.

It all boils down to sensory integration. To know where you are in space, the brain takes in sensory information from multiple systems. These systems include vision, proprioception (for example, information on posture and movement from receptors in the neck), and vestibular input (coming from the inner ear). A person needs each of these senses to provide the brain with information that matches up. When the information from one system does not match up with the others, it causes a sensory mismatch. That is when and why symptoms such as dizziness, vertigo, and disequilibrium can occur.

Sensory integration is something that happens unconsciously. Normally, one never has to think about it. As one moves through the world, the brain just knows exactly where the person is in relationship to their surroundings and knows how the head is moving in relationship to the rest of the body. Losing sense of one's exact position relative to the world can lead to chronic anxiety, a sense of being off-balance, and a sense of feeling disoriented and disconnected from the world around them. Depending on the severity, this can also trigger nausea.

A sensory mismatch situation is like an alarm bell going off in the brain. After even a few seconds of being around a loud alarm, most people feel agitated, irritable, tense, and unable to relax. This is the state of the nervous system when sensory systems are not working together to provide accurate information to the brain on head position and movement.

Key Elements of Sensory Integration

Joint Position Sense

The term "joint position sense" refers to the brain's ability to know what direction a joint is moving, how far, and how fast. The vertebrae, discs, and muscles all contribute to joint position sense of the neck. Trauma to any of these structures or soft tissue in the neck can cause immediate and ongoing alterations of sensory input to the brain, causing a sensory mismatch to take place.

For example, when there is neck trauma and sensory input from the neck is not accurate, it can mean that during head movements, the signal to the brain on how far the head moved may not be accurate. It may also not match up with what the visual system is registering. This sensory mismatch creates confusion in the brain, and for a brief moment, the brain does not accurately register where the head is positioned relative to the rest of the world. This leads to dizziness and a sense of disequilibrium. It can also lead to a persistent sense of neck tension. The brain's unconscious response to a sensory mismatch is often to lock down the neck muscles and minimize head movement, causing pain and stiffness.

Jaw Integration

Imagine a Tyrannosaurus Rex roaring loudly. What is the dinosaur's head doing in this visualization? As it roars, its jaw is opening wide, and its head is rearing backwards.

This is the normal physiology of the jaw. When the jaw opens, neurological reflex pathways going to the back of the neck cause neck extension (but on a much smaller scale than the dinosaur example). Following a TBI, it is very common for people to present in the clinic with a signifi cant amount of jaw tension, in conjunction with neck tension. Together, these can be contributing factors to headaches, disequilibrium, and poor balance.

In my clinic, we quickly assess balance using an iPad application that utilizes the internal gyrometer to detect the degree of movement. By placing acupuncture needles into specific jaw and head muscles involved in jaw opening, testing repeatedly shows that we can achieve immediate improvement in balance with lasting results. Through acupuncture and other therapies, improving sensory integration between the neck and jaw has often led to significant improvements in dizziness, disequilibrium, nausea, headaches, and neck pain in people with these ongoing symptoms following a TBI.

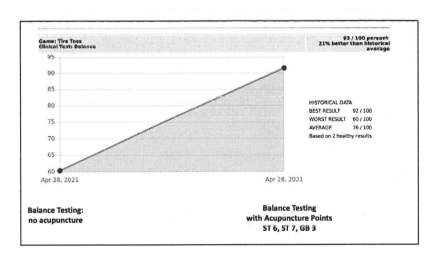

Case Study: Re-establishing Lisa's Sensory Integration

Lisa (name changed for anonymity) came to my office upon the recommendation of another licensed acupuncturist who felt there may be neurological underpinnings to her chronic back pain. Three years prior to seeing me, Lisa had fallen down a flight of stairs and sustained a TBI and fractures in her first cervical vertebra and her seventh, eighth, and ninth thoracic vertebrae.

At 73 years old, Lisa was still working a job requiring a lot of physical activity. She had received regular acupuncture and chiropractic care — specifically, atlas orthogonal treatment. Three years following her injury, her main complaints were neck stiffness, mid-back pain, and muscle spasms. She got temporary relief from her current therapies, but the pain would come back within 24-72 hours. She also had frequent moments of feeling off-balance.

One of the key findings over multiple tests was a left-sided cervical dystonia. Muscles on the left side of her neck were firing inappropriately and were in a chronic state of tension, leading her to have chronic neck pain. I observed this during a head-eye following test, during passive head movements left and right while she fixated her gaze on a center target, and during gait analysis.

When I tested joint position sense of her neck using a laser headlamp device and taking away visual cues, I discovered she wasn't getting accurate feedback from the neck on where it was positioned or how far it was moving. This was likely the cause of a sensory mismatch, resulting in moments of disequilibrium while she was standing and moving.

She also had poor extensor tone on both sides of the body. Extensor muscles allow us to have upright posture and stand easily on two feet. When our neurological pathways involving the vestibular system, cerebellum, and brainstem are working well, standing is easy and not painful. We don't have to consciously fire the muscles allowing us to stand; it happens automatically. In some cases of TBI, these unconscious pathways are affected, and the system ends up recruiting the wrong muscles to fire instead of the normal ones that help us maintain an upright posture. This can lead to chronic back pain and muscle tension or muscle spasms. In Lisa's case, loss of adequate firing of extensor tone pathways caused her back muscles to go into spasm on a regular basis, ending in daily mid-back pain.

The other key finding related directly to Lisa's sense of fatigue during and after work. By the end of her workday, she would feel mentally exhausted, physically in pain, and needed to take a long nap. She didn't have any energy left for anything else. Her job was to assemble online grocery orders for curbside pickup. As she worked her way through the grocery store, she was constantly looking at the order on her phone, then looking at the shelves to find the correct product. All day long, her eyes were darting from near to far to near again. It is very common for a TBI to disrupt normal functioning of these vergence eye movements.

This is exactly what we saw during her exam. More specifically, when she looked from a near target, like her phone, to a far target higher than nose-level, like a top shelf in a grocery store, it was harder than looking from her phone down to a far target that was lower, like a bottom shelf. The difficulty she had with this one specific type of eye movement likely contributed to her occipital pressure and pain, her chronic neck stiffness, and her cognitive fatigue by the end of the day. I identified the specific type of eye movement disorder and most problematic direction by testing vergence eye movements not just from nose-height but also from her right, left, upper, and lower fields of vision. These tests also allowed me to incorporate vergence eye exercises specific to her one area of weakness: looking from her phone to looking at a top shelf in the grocery store hundreds of times a day.

Lisa's treatment plan included cervical spine acupuncture to improve proprioceptive inputs from the neck into the vestibular nucleus in the brainstem, where key aspects of sensory integration occur. After the first treatment of unilateral acupuncture on the left side of her neck, we saw immediate changes in her head-eye following tests, showing a relaxation of the left-sided cervical dystonia. We also included red and infrared light therapy over the three fractured vertebrae in her mid-back, acupuncture along the spine, and myofascial decompression therapies (cupping) on the mid-back.

More importantly, these hands-on therapies were paired with neurological rehab exercises. She was given gaze stabilization exercises, walking head-eye-vestibular retraining exercises, cervical proprioceptive retraining exercises with a laser headlight device, complex off-axis movements helpful for promoting extensor tone, and vergence eye exercises specific to the upper field of vision.

Together, these therapies and exercises helped her brain receive accurate and precise information from her vestibular system, visual system, and cervical proprioceptive system. Her neck muscles relaxed, and her neck pain went away. She was no longer having episodes of disequilibrium. The vergence eye exercises improved eye movements she performed all day long at work. She no longer needed naps at the end of the workday. The pressure in the back of her head went away. Firing up pathways that promoted extensor tone also allowed her mid-back muscles to relax. She no longer had mid-back pain or spasms.

Conclusion

Trauma to the neck can cause many of the same symptoms that are experienced when there is a TBI. Therefore, it is important to address neck injuries in conjunction with TBI rehab. Understanding why neck injuries can cause dizziness, disequilibrium, nausea, and blurry vision involves the concept of sensory integration. Sensory integration, in this context, is the integration of the visual system, vestibular system, and neck proprioceptive system.

A secondary element that should not be ignored is the integration of sensory inputs from jaw muscles into the neck proprioceptive system. Treatment focusing on the neck and jaw can improve sensory integration and have an immediate effect on balance and equilibrium.

As an acupuncturist and Chinese medicine practitioner with additional training in applied clinical neuroscience, I find it essential to combine hands-on therapies, such as acupuncture, with a neurological rehab program tailored to each person's unique clinical presentation.

Dr. Ayla Wolf *is a Doctor of Acupuncture and Oriental Medicine specializing in neurological disorders, chronic pain, and TBI. She is a faculty member of the Carrick Institute. She is an international speaker on topics in applied clinical neuroscience, functional neuroanatomy and neurophysiology, and the biomedical mechanisms of acupuncture. Dr. Wolf is a contributing author to the award-winning book Concussion Discussions: A Functional Approach to Recovery After Brain Injury (Volume 1). During her time in Dallas, Texas, she was the team acupuncturist for the UFC and Legacy fighters training out of Fortis MMA and Octagon. She currently treats patients in her private practice in Stillwater, Minnesota.*

Chapter 3

Identify Post-Concussion Hormone Imbalance with the DUTCH Test

By Dr. Lori Levy, DC, CFMP, CACCP, BA

One of the most challenging aspects of concussion for patients and clinicians is the recovery process. Every patient has questions like: "When will I feel better? When will I be back to normal? When can I do the things that I used to do before?" While physical abilities often get the most attention, biochemical functions usually do not. Things like gastrointestinal function, thyroid health, and hormone health are typically overlooked. Getting a comprehensive hormone assessment following a traumatic brain injury (TBI) could be a key component for the ongoing symptoms you may be suffering.

In a study that compared menstrual patterns of females, 23.5% experienced abnormal menstrual patterns after a head injury, while only 5% with an orthopedic injury had changes in their menstrual cycle.[1] This significant

---

[1] Snook ML, Henry LC, Sanfilippo JS, Zeleznik AJ, Kontos AP. Association of Concussion With Abnormal Menstrual Patterns in Adolescent and Young Women. JAMA Pediatr. 2017 Sep 1;171(9):879-886. doi: 10.1001/jamapediatrics.2017.1140. PMID: 28672284; PMCID: PMC5710410.

finding demonstrates the importance of looking at the deeper structures of the brain that are affected by traumatic injury, including the brain stem and especially the pituitary gland.

The pituitary gland is part of the endocrine system, which includes all of the glands in our bodies that secrete hormones. Like the commander in an army, the pituitary directs the other glands, telling them when to secrete more hormones or when to slow down. It is connected to signals coming from the hypothalamus, also located in the brain. The pituitary tells the thyroid glands to secrete more or less T3 and T4, the ovaries when to secrete more estrogen and progesterone, and the adrenal glands to secrete more or less cortisol, among other functions. The location of the pituitary in the brain predisposes it to injury from a concussion. In fact, up to 37% of patients with TBIs have evidence of low pituitary function within one to five years after their injury.[2]

Although these abnormalities in the endocrine system may take years to be identified, it has been found that various hormones are out of normal ranges even immediately after injury. Elevated levels have been seen in thyroid-stimulating hormone (TSH) and triiodothyronine (T3) as quickly as 48 hours after brain injury, indicating that the hypothalamic-pituitary-thyroid (HPT) axis may be disrupted within the first three days of an injury, which is the acute phase. A disrupted HPT axis can affect thyroid function, potentially causing low energy, weight gain or loss,

---

[2] Di Battista AP, Rhind SG, Churchill N, Richards D, Lawrence DW, Hutchison MG. Peripheral blood neuroendocrine hormones are associated with clinical indices of sport-related concussion. Sci Rep. 2019;9(1):18605. Published 2019 Dec 9. doi:10.1038/s41598-019-54923-3

changes in temperature regulation, and metabolism.

A case series has also shown that blood prolactin levels were suppressed in the acute phase and subsequently elevated throughout recovery.[3] Low prolactin can lead to irregular periods, infertility, breast tenderness, and menopausal symptoms. In the subacute phase, which starts around four days post-injury and can last up to six weeks, abnormally low blood cortisol levels were seen, which were associated with increased post-TBI symptoms and longer recovery time.[4] Low cortisol can cause fatigue, dizziness (especially when standing up), muscle weakness, and mood changes.

Both men and women were shown to have significantly altered hormone levels after a severe TBI, including increased estradiol in men and increased testosterone in women.[5] What is even more interesting is that women may be more susceptible to subsequent endocrine complications if the injury occurs at a certain time of their menstrual cycle.[6]

The menstrual cycle has two different phases: the follicular phase, making up the first 14 days, and the luteal

[3] La Fountaine MF, Toda M, Testa A, Bauman WA. Suppression of Serum Prolactin Levels after Sports Concussion with Prompt Resolution Upon Independent Clinical Assessment To Permit Return-to-Play. J Neurotrauma. 2016;33:904–906. doi: 10.1089/neu.2015.3968.

[4] Ritchie EV, Emery C, Debert CT. Analysis of serum cortisol to predict recovery in paediatric sport-related concussion. Brain Inj. 2018;32:523–528. doi: 10.1080/02699052.2018.1429662.

[5] Wagner AK, McCullough EH, Niyonkuru C, Ozawa H, Loucks TL, Dobos JA, Brett CA, Santarsieri M, Dixon CE, Berga SL, Fabio A. Acute serum hormone levels: characterization and prognosis after severe traumatic brain injury. J Neurotrauma. 2011 Jun;28(6):871-88. doi: 10.1089/neu.2010.1586. Epub 2011 Jun 1. PMID: 21488721; PMCID: PMC3113446.

[6] Wunderle K, Hoeger KM, Wasserman E, Bazarian JJ. Menstrual phase as predictor of outcome after mild traumatic brain injury in women. J Head Trauma Rehabil. 2014;29(5):E1-E8. doi:10.1097/HTR.0000000000000006

phase, making up the second 14 days. The luteal phase is when progesterone concentration is highest. Progesterone is a hormone that has neuroprotective effects, which reduces brain swelling when administered after injury for up to 24 hours.[7] When comparing quality of life outcome measures 30 days after the injury, women in the luteal phase, when progesterone is highest, had worse outcomes than women in the follicular phase of their cycle, when progesterone is lowest. This is because the injury caused such a drop in progesterone that the brain suffered from the loss of neuroprotective effects.

It is likely that the impact of trauma to the head affects the neuroendocrine system in a way similar to how it affects the thyroid and adrenals: causing a significant drop in hormone levels. Specifically, drops in progesterone have been documented, taking away its neuroprotective effects. The drop in hormones following a TBI may explain why women frequently miss menstrual periods or experience a complete loss of their menstrual cycle. If progesterone continues to be depressed, then headaches, anxiety, forgetfulness, and mood changes may occur since there may be lower levels found in the brain. Though it may be assumed that these hormones do not affect men, men make these hormones as well, and there can be negative consequences when they are imbalanced.

In my practice, one of the lab tests I use for assessing hormones is the DUTCH Plus test, which stands for Dried Urine Test for Comprehensive Hormones. Unlike typical hormone testing, which is done via blood, the DUTCH

---

[7] Singh M, Su C. Progesterone and neuroprotection. Horm Behav. 2013;63(2):284-290. doi:10.1016/j.yhbeh.2012.06.003

tests hormones in urine and saliva. It is one of the most comprehensive looks we can get when it comes to hormones. It is extremely helpful because not only are hormone levels measured, but how we are processing them is also measured. So while testing hormones in serum can be helpful, the DUTCH Plus test looks at overall hormone levels in addition to different metabolites in urine and saliva, telling us if you are processing hormones in beneficial or harmful ways, if they are being cleared out of the system, and in what ratios they are being cleared.

In comparison with most blood tests for hormones which typically assess only estradiol (E2), the DUTCH test looks at even more than that. When it comes to estrogen, it can be a very generic term, and most of the time it refers to estradiol. On the DUTCH test, there are three forms of estrogen levels assessed: estrone (E1), estradiol (E2), and estriol (E3), in addition to how they get processed in the body. The most potent of these, and the most commonly referred to, is estradiol. However, E1 and E3 contribute to total estrogen as well, making it important to assess all three.

Other hormone markers on the DUTCH test include:
1.   alpha-pregnanediol
2.   beta-pregnanediol
3.   DHEA
4.   DHEA-S
5.   androsterone
6.   etiocholanone
7.   5-a-DHT
8.   5-a-androstanediol
9.   5-b-androstanediol

10.   epi-testosterone

What can't be seen in a blood test for hormones are metabolites of hormones, meaning how the hormones are getting processed by the body. This can only be seen on a urine test. The body has a system of processing or detoxing hormones, similar to how machines process trash or recycling. This detoxification pathway includes a phase 1 and phase 2 system in the liver, which can be assessed using the DUTCH test.

Markers included to assess phase 1 and 2 detoxification pathways include:

- 2-OH-E1
- 4-OH-E1
- 16-OH-E1
- 2-Methoxy-E1
- 2-OH-E2
- 4-OH-E2

It is important to know not only how much of these metabolites are being made, but also what the ratio of those metabolites are. This tells us if the body can keep up with clearing out excess hormones. Your body also relies on the ability to do phase 1 clearing to continue detoxification into phase 2, which is the final punch through the liver to get the estrogen cleared up and moved out of the body.

Estrogen metabolites have different properties; therefore, making too much of one and not enough of another can be harmful to the body. Think of them as the good, the bad, and the ugly. The good is the 2-OH, where you want to push most of your estrogen down and is a protective form of estrogen. Between 60-80% of estrogen should be sent down this pathway. The bad is the 4-OH, which can create health issues if it gets too high. We only want approximately 7-11% of estrogen going down this pathway. If it exceeds that, it can cause damage to DNA and potentially contribute to the development of breast cancer. The ugly is the 16-OH, which has some good properties that protect bone health and some bad properties that can create fibrocystic breast problems. Sending between 13-30% of estrogen down this pathway is expected.

The total estrogen values can then be assessed along with progesterone to determine if there is balance between the two hormones. Even with a "normal range" of progesterone, excessive amounts of estrogen will create a physiologic state that mimics that of low lab value of progesterone. This is referred to as "relative" estrogen dominance. This could also contribute to irregular menstrual cycles after a TBI.

Similar to estrogen metabolites, the DUTCH test also assesses metabolites of progesterone. Your body makes alpha-pregnanediol and beta-pregnanediol. Sometimes, your body has a preference for making one or the other, which can also be seen on the DUTCH test. Alpha-pregnanediol is considered neuroprotective. It can cross the blood brain barrier and increase a neurotransmitter called GABA, which is very calming and decreases anxiety. This could be beneficial as it can create a sense of calm and help with sleep. If your body has a drop in progesterone due to a TBI, the opposite could be the case.

The DUTCH test also assesses the cortisol awakening response through saliva, which is a key indicator in evaluating the hypothalamic-pituitary-adrenal (HPA) axis. The HPA axis refers to interaction/communication between the hypothalamus and pituitary in the brain down to the adrenal glands that sit on top of your kidneys. When the body needs cortisol, the hypothalamus releases cortisol-releasing hormone (CRH), and the pituitary responds by releasing adrenocorticotropic hormone (ACTH), which is the signal to the adrenal gland to release cortisol, DHEA, and DHEA-S. These adrenal hormones are all assessed on the DUTCH test in an effort to understand the patient's HPA axis. This is a key thing to assess if you have a brain injury, and it's often overlooked.

If you have experienced a TBI and have continued to experience hormone-related symptoms, know that they are connected. The force to your brain has more effects than is often accounted for in your medical assessments, and blood testing can only give you so much information. The DUTCH test can give you a more detailed picture of what is happening with your hormones and how they are being processed, and can help you treat short-term symptoms and avoid long-term problems.

Dr. Lori Levy *(formerly Dr. Lori Jokinen) earned her Doctor of Chiropractic degree from Northwestern Health Sciences University, graduating with cum laude honors. She holds a certification from the Academy Council of Chiropractic Pediatrics and is a certified functional medicine practitioner. Dr. Lori is currently completing her diplomate degree in Clinical Nutrition. She is also certified in acupuncture and Graston technique. Dr. Lori Levy completed her undergraduate education at the University of Minnesota, earning a Bachelor of Arts degree in psychology.*

Chapter 4

Searching for the Right Questions: The Role of the Brainstem in Post-Concussive POTS

By Mehul Parekh, DC, DACNB

On a Monday morning in May 2021, I met Annie and her mother Lisa for the first time. I had been in contact with Lisa for several months regarding her daughter's long-standing health conditions. In December 2015, a then-11-year-old Annie was knocked unconscious when she hit her head against a tree while sledding down a steep hill near her home in Montana. Within the next six months, she gradually began displaying a variety of disparate symptoms. Separately, Annie was diagnosed with three conditions: postural orthostatic tachycardia syndrome (POTS), Ehlers-Danlos syndrome (EDS), and mast cell activation syndrome (MCAS).

The next few years saw Annie, Lisa, and the rest of their family traveling around the country looking for answers and struggling to find them. Though all of these symptoms began in the immediate aftermath of a head injury, this was dismissed as a potential cause for what Annie experienced on a daily basis. Their family's health history and the established understanding that all three of these conditions have some root in genetics suggested that there was no reason why Annie was dealing with all of this, and her doctors set out to manage her symptoms individually as best they could. By the time Annie arrived at Northwest Functional Neurology (NWFN) in Portland, Oregon, she had also recently dealt with a COVID-19 infection, which only served to worsen her existing symptoms.

A Triad of Conditions

At first glance, you may look at these three diagnoses and wonder what they are — and what on earth they have in common.

POTS refers to a disorder in which blood is unable to appropriately return from the feet to the midline when standing up. It is categorized as a form of dysautonomia, which describes an inability to regulate the autonomic nervous system. What sets POTS apart is the well-defined diagnostic criteria — an increase in heart rate of at least 30 beats per minute when moving from laying flat to standing up, and a standing heart rate of over 120 beats per minute.

EDS refers to a disorder of the body's connective tissue. This can present in several different ways, but among the more common presentations, we see joint hypermobility, excessive skin elasticity, or a lack of appropriate collagen within the walls of arteries. This lack of collagen impedes the arteries' contractile properties, so when blood pumps to the feet, the arteries lack the proper peripheral resistance, which, as an immediate consequence, leads to orthostatic hypotension — a drop in blood pressure when standing up. What's more, as more blood pools in the feet, the heart has to pump faster to generate proper circulation.

MCAS describes improper levels of activity of the immune cells that govern our allergic response. Mast cells are capable of releasing any of over 200 chemicals in response to signals from the immune system. MCAS, however, is a condition where mast cells spring into action without immune system signaling. Patients can experience the type of symptoms we would associate with any allergic reaction, be it congestion, intense gastrointestinal (GI) symptoms, or even anaphylactic shock.

The challenges in dealing with these conditions are significant. For one, the conditions themselves present in ways that defy our current understanding of them. From there, the relationships among these three conditions are not well-defined or easily understood. In fact, some research dismisses the idea of a causative link altogether. Other research has tried to identify enzymes and proteins that are present in at least two of the three conditions. Currently, some research has indicated that as many as 31 percent of patients with MCAS may also suffer from POTS and EDS.

Treating this triad is truly a team effort. And our role within that team was to look at the entirety of Annie and ask enough questions to determine our best way forward.

Annie's Examination

Our first step in determining how to best help Annie was taking a detailed history. Soon after her accident, Annie initially experienced headaches and neck pain, which were not surprising given the nature and severity of her injury. However, she also noticed joint pain throughout her body in areas not directly impacted by the collision. She began feeling dizzy and light-headed on a daily basis, to the point where standing up caused her to feel like she was about to black out. When she could stay standing without these blackout sensations, she noticed rapid pooling of blood in her feet. Even five years later, when we were treating her, these blackout episodes occurred daily.

As if that was not enough, Annie began dealing with intense stomach pain, feelings of chronic nausea, and reduced appetite. She also began having episodes of full-body breakouts of hives and cheeks that looked and felt sunburned. All of these symptoms conspired to hospitalize Annie by the summer of 2016 due to rapid weight loss — at age 12, her weight dropped to under 80 pounds. She needed an IV cocktail of Benadryl, Zyrtec, and anti-nausea and anxiety medications every six hours just to make it through the day.

We followed Annie's history with a battery of cutting-edge diagnostic testing. We performed computerized posturography to evaluate her balance in a variety of circumstances, video nystagmography (VNG) to evaluate her eye movements, and head-impulse testing to determine the quality and integrity of her vestibular-ocular reflexes.

Finally, we performed a detailed physical examination, which allowed us to take a detailed look at her cognitive, physical, neurological, and autonomic functioning. This included a tilt table evaluation, for which Annie lay flat on a table which was gradually elevated in five- to ten-degree increments. At each increment, we evaluated her blood pressure and heart rate. Our goal was to find an inflection point at which her brain and brainstem could not effectively regulate her blood flow to her extremities and back to her brain. It only took 25 degrees' worth of elevation for Annie's heart rate, already high at a baseline of 99 beats per minute, to elevate to 121. It was no wonder Annie frequently felt like she was going to black out when standing up! This sudden and dramatic increase in heart rate met the clearly defined parameters for POTS.

The Brainstem

The entirety of the first day's process is about outlining areas that need rehabilitation. One of the primary areas we identified was the brainstem. Think of the brainstem as the stalk holding up the cortex (a head of broccoli) on top of it. When someone suffers a hit like Annie, they deal with simultaneous forces hitting their head and neck from multiple angles. This leads to the head of broccoli bouncing back and forth, which is what many people typically envision in a mild traumatic brain injury (TBI).

Beyond that, the stalk underneath the head gets shaken around as well. These multi-directional force vectors have the highest degree of impact in the lower brainstem, which is comprised of two parts: the pons and the medulla oblongata. In any post-concussive case, rehabilitation of the lower brainstem is a critical component. This is an area involved in eye movement, gaze stabilization, descending pain modulation pathways, and control of resting muscle tone, among other things.

The PPRF

The lower brainstem houses areas that are critical in understanding how we could best help Annie's recovery. The first area to identify is the pontine paramedian reticular formation (PPRF). The PPRF receives input from various areas within the brainstem and cortex and is directly involved in generating a specific class of eye movements called saccades. Saccades are defined as rapid, self-directed eye movements from one visual target to another. When we evaluate these eye movements, we look at four characteristics:

1. Latency, or time needed to initiate the saccade
2. Velocity of the eye movement from the first target to the next
3. Accuracy of the eyes in mapping out the target
4. Stability of visual gaze fixation once the eyes arrive at the target

The pathways associated with saccade generation are complex, too complex for a brief discussion here. But it is important to understand that while they are seen as an indicator of frontal lobe health, appropriate saccades require all aspects of the neuraxis to be properly calibrated, and the lower brainstem is chief among these areas. It is also important to note that research has borne out that at least one, if not all four, of the quantifiable characteristics of saccades can be affected by brain injury.

The PPRF houses two distinct classes of neurons: burst and pause. Think of these burst and pause neurons as having a gas-and-brake relationship that allows us to jump our eyes to a target when we need to, not just at random. This is critical to helping us understand where visual targets are in our world and how to find them efficiently. In a TBI, it is common to see either the gas firing too high or the brakes keeping the eyes stuck.

Other Lower Brainstem Regions

Beyond its role in eye movement generation, the PPRF directly modulates two other critical lower brainstem regions. One is called the NTS, or nucleus tractus solitarius. The NTS sits at the junction of the pons and medulla and directly projects to the carotid artery to regulate the stretch of arteries throughout the system. This is the first step in how the brainstem monitors peripheral blood flow and commands the arteries to either further constrict or dilate, depending on the rest of the body's need for proper blood supply.

The lower brainstem also houses the dorsal motor nucleus of vagus nerve (DMNV), a cranial nerve that affects the functioning of every internal organ. The vagus nerve supplies signals to the heart's built-in electrochemical regulatory system, ensuring healthy heart rate and rhythm. From there, the vagus nerve has a direct effect on several GI functions, such as gut motility. When normal GI activity is decreased, some of Annie's symptoms (nausea, bloating, difficulty with digestion) are to be expected. But the level of discomfort she experienced, coupled with a reliance on antihistamines, speaks to the intersection of gut dysbiosis and MCAS. It is difficult to separate where one condition ends and the other begins, but the best way to think of it is this: Annie's immune system was primed for this, and her TBI released the hounds.

Annie's Treatment

It was clear that lower brainstem rehabilitation was going to be a component of Annie's rehabilitation. The next question was: What was the best approach?

Through our diagnostic testing, we were able to identify which areas needed to be rehabilitated, but which pathways were the most viable and could be beneficial in the recovery process? Within the VNG exam, we took a detailed look at Annie's ability to generate saccades in a variety of circumstances. Annie's mapping of her visual field showed notable aberrancies, and these only worsened as we tested her endurance by having her saccade back and forth between two set targets for several minutes. As we tested her endurance, her latency began to slightly increase, indicating a propensity for fatigue. She also struggled to hold her eyes steady at visual targets.

Additionally, Annie's rightward saccade accuracy progressively worsened as testing ensued, as did her ability to fixate on saccade targets. The combination of these two greatly distorted her sense of where she was in space. She experienced a sensory mismatch in her insular and cingulate cortices, areas of the brain responsible for body mapping, processing of sensory information from the inner ear and body and modulating the autonomic nervous system. These areas have some margin for error; an occasional unstable or inaccurate eye movement does not throw our world into chaos. But when we repeatedly demonstrate an inability to map out our world and make sense of where the visual environment is and where we fit in it, the cingulate cortex sounds a five alarm error response throughout our brain.

This stress response leads to immediate brainstem dysregulation and disinhibition of the sympathetic nervous system. We begin to perspire, our pupils dilate, our GI system slows to a crawl, and our peripheral nervous system lowers its resistance to increased blood flow, leading to decreased blood pressure. Heart rate increases, and the inability to map our bodies leads to impaired blood flow back to the midline, which only feeds into this cycle of orthostatic hypotension and tachycardia. In short, Annie's inability to appropriately shift her eyes from one target to another directly escalated her collection of symptoms. Rehabilitating this pathway was intrinsic to her recovery.

But it was not all bad news — in fact, much of the news was quite positive. Annie's initial latencies were not only in a normal range, but were optimal for a 17-year-old. Latency is an established representation of a system's plasticity — that is, its ability to rebuild appropriate synaptic connections throughout the neuraxis. Though they were prone to fatigue, Annie's saccade latencies remained largely stable. This demonstrated that her potential for improvement was significant. With all this information at our disposal, we set about creating a path towards recovery.

Annie spent two weeks with us at NWFN as part of our NeuroRescue intensive rehabilitation program. We customized a program of brain rehab exercises, electrical stimulation, sensorimotor integrative exercises, and restorative therapies aimed at stabilizing and rehabilitating her brainstem pathways. We worked at a level of intensity and duration that was carefully designed to avoid causing unnecessary fatigue. Every two to three days, Annie repeated diagnostic testing. Based on her results, we modified her treatment protocol to further focus on the particular pathways in most need of rehabilitation.

Annie completed her two-week protocol in May 2021, and she returned for a three-day follow-up a few months later. Her diagnostics have shown that her saccade functioning has improved significantly — not only are her eyes stable at targets, but she no longer struggles with visual mapping and accuracy. Her latency has remained optimal and is no longer susceptible to the level of fatigue it was before.

Annie has reported a significant reduction in the frequency of her blackout episodes. Three days into her intensive, she was able to eat a chicken sandwich without intense nausea, and she was able to sit through a friend's softball game without feeling like she was going to fall over. She no longer has to wear compression stockings throughout the day to control the pooling of blood in her feet. Her resting heart rate now generally sits in the mid-70s, and she can stand up out of bed without getting immediately dizzy.

Continued Progress

With all that said, Annie's rehabilitation is a work in progress. We have co-managed her MCAS and EDS with other providers, and we have taken a deep dive into aspects of her neuroimmunology through detailed lab testing. Each of her diagnoses individually posed challenges, and the understanding of the intersection of POTS, EDS, and MCAS is still being explored. While I would love to tell you that Annie is 100 percent fixed, the truth is, her condition will require long-term monitoring, starting with detailed research and progressing to medical innovation.

But through it all, Annie and Lisa recognize that she has made more progress in two weeks with us, and the home exercises and follow-up afterward, than in the five years prior. More than anything, they both feel that our approach has given them some measurable and quantifiable information that has helped them make sense of Annie's unique challenges.

More than providing all of the answers, we are happy that we were able to ask the right questions, and together with Annie and Lisa, put her puzzle together and come up with some solutions that help her regain some measure of freedom from a challenging condition. Our results with Annie have compelled Lisa to become a patient herself, to better identify the biomarkers underlying her neurological concerns.

Lisa starts with us soon. And we will aim to ask the right questions again.

Dr. Mehul Parekh received his undergraduate degrees from the University of Rochester and the State University of New York: College at Brockport, where he graduated summa cum laude in exercise physiology. From there, he studied at Life University in Marietta, Georgia, earning his Doctor of Chiropractic degree in 2015. He has been recognized by the American Chiropractic Neurology Board as a board-certified chiropractic neurologist since

2016. Since 2019, he has been a chiropractic physician at Northwest Functional Neurology.

Chapter 5

Concussions and the Importance of Balance

By Dr. Michael Schmidt, DC, DACNB

Balance, according to Cambridge Dictionary, is "the condition of someone or something in which its weight is equally divided so that it can stay in one position or be under control while moving."

Our independence depends upon balance and being able to stand and walk around, yet we take for granted our ability to maintain adequate balance in different conditions. When we are an infant and our brain is developing, we are unable to walk and maintain balance. As we age and our brain deteriorates or we obtain a concussion or traumatic brain injury, once again we lose the ability to maintain balance and will make use of a cane or wheelchair.

Balance or posture is achieved through the brain's correct integration of information coming from three systems: your eyes/vision, the muscles and joints of your body, and your vestibular inner ear balance system — along with a coordinated motor activity or response, which is dependent upon muscle strength, accuracy, and speed of response to your environment. What this means is after a concussion or brain injury, if either one of those three sensory systems or the brain areas that control them have been hurt or are not communicating and integrating with the other two, there will be a loss of balance. All three have to be working together like an orchestra.

Symptoms of Loss of Balance

Let's discuss symptoms related to these three sensory systems. Keep in mind that they are just that — symptoms. They seldom point to where the real problem is, but along with a great neurological exam, they can help at getting to the bottom of your balance issues.

After a concussion, some primary eye/visual symptoms could involve double vision, blurry vision, eye pain or strain, headaches, fogginess, and/or loss of depth perception, causing a loss of balance. These could be due to the eye/visual areas of the brain being injured, or it could even be due to the wrong information coming from the other two areas (muscles/joints and vestibular system) as they have to work together.

Symptoms following a concussion involving primarily muscles and joints include trouble standing on one leg, inability to walk in a straight line, feeling uncoordinated or clumsy, and frequent falls while standing or walking, especially when it is dark out. Yet again, this could be due to this specific area being damaged, but one of the other two systems could be involved as well.

Symptoms that someone could experience that involve primarily the vestibular system are dizziness, nausea, lightheadedness, feeling like you are floating, and vertigo, which is when the room feels like it's moving or you feel like you are moving when you are still. All of these symptoms can be made worse by turning your head or neck too fast. Again, this could be due to this specific brain area being injured and/or could have involvement from the other two systems.

Balance Testing

Someone who has had a concussion or is currently suffering from post-concussion symptoms such as these should be evaluated by a trained functional neurologist or a chiropractic neurologist. The evaluation involves looking into detail at all three of these systems and how well they are working together.

During the actual examination, numerous other testing and diagnostics are used to evaluate all areas of the brain and body, but we will focus on balance, including different testing conditions and potential treatment scenarios. If you have had a concussion and are suffering from a loss of balance or are wondering if you have a loss of balance, I encourage you to try some of these at home in a safe area so that you can catch yourself if you lose balance.

Step one of the evaluation is measuring heart rate, blood pressure, and oxygen saturation while you are lying down, seated, and then standing to ensure you can regulate your vitals in all positions. We are especially looking for any significant amount of increase or decrease in the heart rate or blood pressure when going from lying to seated or seated to standing, as that is abnormal and can contribute to a loss of balance.

Static Balance Tests

The next important step is diving into detail with balance testing. The first condition tested is typically static balance, which means you are standing as still as you can in different conditions. Different levels of difficulty would include feet spaced apart with eyes open then closed, feet together with eyes open then closed, on a foam pad (you can use a solid pillow instead) with eyes open then closed, tandem stance (one foot directly in front of the other) with eyes open then closed, and a single-leg stance with eyes open then closed.

An abnormal result in a static balance test would be if you feel any symptoms or an increase in symptoms, or if you lose balance by taking a step, swaying a lot, or throwing your arms out to stabilize. A functional neurologist would also check for a neck and eye component; we would have you tilt your head in different directions and hold it there while maintaining balance, with your eyes open then closed. Then, we would have you hold your eyes in different directions — left/right, up/down, and diagonal — while holding balance. Any increase in sway, loss of balance, or increase in symptoms or new symptoms would be considered abnormal and would tell us that your eyes, neck, and/or vestibular system could be involved in your loss of balance.

Dynamic Balance Tests

The second condition tested is dynamic balance, which means we are trying to see how well you can balance while moving or performing an activity.

As a physician, I like to start this one with your feet together, looking straight ahead, and have you follow my thumb with your eyes going left/right, up/down, and diagonally while I look for a loss of balance or a return of symptoms. Then, you would turn your head left to right and then up and down, with your eyes open then closed, and if needed, we would move to a foam pad to check these once again. Again, an abnormal test result would be losing balance, putting an arm out to brace, taking a step, or an increase in current symptoms or new symptoms. Any of these would indicate that the eyes, neck, and/or vestibular system are involved with your balance issues.

Up next for dynamic balance is testing your limit of stability (LOS). Stand with either your feet together or slightly apart and your arms to your sides, keeping your body as straight as you can. Then, lean your entire body — almost like a tower — in different directions: left and right, forwards and backwards, and diagonally. What we are looking for here is that you can lean in all these different directions without throwing your hands up, taking a step, or getting symptoms, and also how far you are able to lean in these different directions.

The next set of dynamic balance tests add in reaching tasks. First, put your feet together and reach your arms out forwards, to the sides, and backwards. Then, reach a foot forward while balancing on one leg, and then gradually move your foot to the side. You can also stand on a foam pad and perform the same foot exercise. With these specific dynamic balance tests, there is usually a specific direction that causes more swaying, a feeling of instability or loss of balance, or a return of symptoms, which tells us if the arms or legs are involved with your loss of balance. Some extra dynamic balance tests include trying to walk a line forwards and backwards, performing with eyes open then eyes closed, and then marching in place while doing the same thing.

If you do these tests at home and notice that you are very unstable, unable to complete a test, or feel symptoms during a test, then you should contact your nearest functional neurologist and allow them to assist you. A functional neurologist will most likely have a balance platform to test all of the aforementioned tests and will be able to compare your data to a normative data range for your age and gender, giving you even more detailed results.

As you can see, there is a progression to the testing — as well as to the therapy that would then be applied. Knowing where to start is most important when it comes to treating balance, and a trained functional neurologist will know exactly where to start based on your balance testing results.

Balance Therapy

The treatments or therapies used to improve balance are very similar to the tests, but we can gear them toward the areas that need the most help or that showed the most abnormal test results.

Functional neurologists keep an eye out for fatigue during your treatments and therapies. It is very important to not push past fatigue, as it will be detrimental to the healing process. Just like at the gym, you cannot curl 50 pounds without starting at a lower weight and increasing it over time.

If you had a significant loss of balance when you were following a target with your eyes or when you were holding your eyes in different directions, that points to an involvement of your visual/eye system. A trained functional neurologist may do individualized eye movement training, starting seated or lying down and eventually working toward standing in all of the different balance conditions until you do not have symptoms or lose balance.

If your balance was substantially worse with your eyes closed in a majority of the testing, the areas and pathways of your brain that control your muscles and joints are not working as well as they should. Your doctor may do different types of massage, soft tissue work, chiropractic manipulations, or even body exercises. They may also have you practice balancing in different conditions with your eyes closed, progressing only when you don't feel symptoms or lose your balance.

If your balance worsened significantly in all of the tests that involved moving your neck and head, that points to an issue with your neck muscles and joints or with the vestibular system. Your doctor may provide stretches, soft tissue work, massage, exercises, and chiropractic manipulations to the neck, along with specific vestibular-based exercises starting seated or lying down and moving to standing, each involving different neck and head movements.

Conclusion

If you have had a concussion or brain injury and have problems with balance, it is important to see a trained functional neurologist, who will complete a thorough examination as well as balance testing. Although you can complete balance tests at home, a functional neurologist can prescribe the appropriate treatments and therapies for your particular condition. With patience and consistent practice, your balance will improve, lowering the risk of further brain injuries from falls and allowing you to move more freely — perhaps even helping you reclaim your independence.

Dr. Michael Schmidt, DC, DACNB grew up on a farm in Centralia, Missouri, playing sports, including baseball, football, and wrestling. Upon graduating high school, he received a scholarship to wrestle at the University of Missouri (MU) in Columbia. After four years at MU, he graduated with a Bachelor's of Science in Health Sciences. He then attended Logan University in St. Louis, receiving his Doctorate of Chiropractic in 2017. Dr. Schmidt received post-graduate training in vestibular rehabilitation, traumatic brain injury (TBI), childhood developmental disorders, functional medicine, and functional neurology. He was honored with receiving diplomate status from the American Chiropractic Neurology Board in 2017. He aims to spread awareness of functional neurology's ability to use a brain-based approach in helping traditional chiropractic patients, patients with concussions and TBIs, and patients with neurological conditions.

Chapter 6

Learning How to Walk after COVID, as Featured on ABC News

By Dr. Marc Ellis D.C. MS, NMT, DACNB, FACFN, FABBIR

Afsheen Ali was living a pleasant life in 2020 as a successful businesswoman and mother in Homewood, Alabama, when her life was impacted by COVID-19. She contracted and seemingly recovered from the virus, but nothing could have prepared her for the after-effects.

No one at this time was talking about the crippling physical ramifications Afsheen was experiencing. The terms "post-COVID syndrome" and "long-haulers syndrome" had yet to enter our vernacular. After three weeks of quarantine, she thought she was doing better, but she was unable to walk or feel her legs. Her problem was compounded by chronic fatigue and difficulty breathing.

Afsheen went to the University of Alabama's post-COVID clinic and several doctors, to no avail. She said it appeared no one seemed to understand what was happening to her. Some doctors told her it was "all in her head" and that she needed a positive mental attitude. She did everything she could to get better, but she could not walk without assistance.

ABC News did a report on Afsheen and her treatment at our clinic. She told ABC News, "I'm not myself anymore and don't know when I'll get it back. Nobody gets it. What's the problem? On the outside, I look fine, but on the inside, I am so broken, so shaken."[8]

It is now well known that chronic post-COVID symptoms can affect numerous body systems, including the nervous, cardiovascular, pulmonary, endocrine, immune, and musculoskeletal systems. Due to the novelty of this condition, physicians are still learning how to treat patients. Afsheen was referred to me at the Georgia Chiropractic Neurology Center by her friend who is also a chiropractor and is familiar with my work.

A Physical Examination Changes Afsheen's Life

Afsheen came to our office accompanied by her husband. She was confined to a wheelchair and said her feet were extremely cold, numb, and heavy, and that they felt like solid blocks of ice. She was so convinced her feet were cold, she thought I would be able to feel the temperature change through her shoes. She also reported brain fog, short-term memory issues, sensitivity to light, and heaviness of her head.

---

[8] Gould, Cynthia. COVID long hauler now walking again, says recovery was 'nothing short of a miracle.' ABC News. 22 March 2021. https://abc3340.com/news/abc-3340-news-iteam/covid-longhauler-now-walking-again-says-recovery-was-nothing-short-of-a-miracle

A Helpful Diagnosis

An in-depth neurological examination revealed that Afsheen had a normal ability to feel different sensations, such as sharp, dull, and vibration, and she was able to move her limbs in all directions. However, she was unable to walk despite having full range of motion and function.

I diagnosed this as limb-kinetic apraxia. Apraxias are conditions where the person cannot correctly perform a learned movement like walking or combing their hair, but they have normal sensations and can perform other movements. These patients appear to have problems in higher brain centers that can affect certain types of movements.

Afsheen had difficulty being able to sense where her legs and feet were, which I assessed by performing a frequently overlooked test called single-point localization. In this test, the examiner has the patient close their eyes and then touch the body part in question. The patient is instructed to touch where the doctor is touching. Afsheen could not accurately locate where she was being touched on her lower legs and feet.

It is essential for a person to know where their leg is in order to then be able to move it. If the brain cannot accurately interpret and integrate messages that are coming from the body, they will not move correctly. This can manifest as repetitive sprain or strain injuries, muscle weakness, or decreased coordination. For Afsheen, it was more extreme and stifled her ability to walk.

An Astute Observation: Abnormally Low Temperatures

Another important finding for her specific situation was a change in the temperature of her legs and feet. Her lower leg was 85°F, her foot was 73°F, and her toes were 71°F. She was surprised because they felt much colder than that, but she was also relieved because someone was able to measure her temperature change and understand her situation.

An Astute Observation: Dyssynchronization of the Brain

Afsheen and her husband were working hard to comprehend the situation. They had brain MRIs, EEGs, and other exam findings that led doctors to tell them nothing was wrong. But if nothing was wrong, why could she no longer walk? Why had she lost her self-sufficiency? She could no longer work, drive, or take care of her family.

I explained the similarity between a concussion and her condition caused from the virus affecting her brain. She had dyssynchronization in brain areas that were related to walking, which in turn gave her dysautonomia: poor functioning of her autonomic nervous system. In Afsheen's case, dysautonomia presented as poor regulation of temperature and blood flow in her feet.

Afsheen and her husband finally felt a sense of relief because after a year of searching, someone explained her situation in a way that made sense and gave them hope that she could actually regain her quality of life.

Pinpointing the Correct Treatments

Afsheen had already been to physical therapy for walking and vestibular rehab — with little to no improvement. I used a NeXus-10 biofeedback system to monitor the temperature in her toes and started with conservative eye tracking and movement therapies via the Interactive Metronome. I observed that both of these treatments caused the temperature in her legs and feet to drop.

The fundamental theory in functional neurology is to monitor physiological responses. It quickly became evident that these therapies triggered an increase in the sympathetic nervous system and caused the circulation to become diminished to muscles of the foot and leg and to correlating areas of the central nervous system, brain, and spinal cord. I immediately knew that while these treatments are beneficial for other patients, they were not for Afsheen; she needed different therapies.

I shifted Afsheen's care plan and implemented single-point localization therapies to improve her body awareness. These therapies resulted in improved temperature in her feet and legs. I monitored her temperature, and when it would drop, she would rest until she was ready for more treatments. Once she regained an accurate awareness of her feet, she was able to stand without the use of her walker. She commented that for the first time in months, she could feel her feet, and the sensation that they were encased in ice was gone.

By the end of the first day, the temperature in her toes increased from 71°F to 75°F. This small step forward (no pun intended) was very encouraging to her! It is very common that when treating patients in these challenging situations, any step forward is good. And like so many other people, she had more steps forward that she was about to achieve.

Now, Afsheen was ready to integrate how she saw her body in relationship to where she saw her world. I accomplished this by adding a therapy where dots were lined up in a row on her body, and the last dot was placed on her lower leg. She looked from dot to dot until she reached the one on her leg and then touched it.

One of the most important areas for visual maps is in the brainstem. It's called the superior colliculus, and it sends messages to the parietal lobe and affects regions of the brain for self-awareness. The relationship between these two brain regions is essential for organizing your body's world-orientation to your self-orientation. Failure of these systems to align can have dire consequences and create situations where you feel disoriented and lose your ability to move correctly.

Vision therapy that calibrates your world to your body returns proper relationship between these brain areas, thereby allowing you to regain your ability to move. For Afsheen, this was a critical treatment. Her temperature increased to 84°F in her shins and 78°F in her feet and toes. By the end of the third day, she was able to walk six steps without assistance.

A Sure Step Forward

When Afsheen arrived at the office for the fourth day of care, she had turned a corner (again, no pun intended!).

Her body had finally begun the innate process of self-healing. She maintained her ability to walk a few steps, and her temperature improved overnight to 88°F in the shin and 83°F in the feet and toes.

Afsheen's condition and seven months of being wheelchair-bound had caused her to no longer know how to correctly shift her weight to move or walk. I used a tool called the Comprehensive Assessment of Postural Systems (CAPS) and designed a program for her. Afsheen would stand on a force plate while targets appeared on a television screen in patterns that I had specifically programmed for her. She would shift her weight, and the force plate would measure her location in relationship to the target. She could see if she was accurate or not on the TV and would adjust her weight until she could hit the targets.

After two more days of care, Afsheen regained her ability to walk normally. She could finally care for her family and return to work again.

Conclusion

Doctors at our clinic have helped thousands of patients with COVID long-haulers symptoms. The pandemic has affected the lives of countless people, but not all in the same way. The neurological symptoms of post-COVID syndrome include brain fog, headache, sleep problems, dizziness, and POTS, which stands for postural orthostatic tachycardia syndrome and affects blood flow. Other patients suffer from fatigue, light and sound sensitivity, and loss of smell and taste. Many patients report feelings of tingling in different parts of their body or various types of joint pain. We have also treated many brain-injured patients over the years who have suffered from apraxia.

Afsheen was unique in that her apraxia appeared after she had COVID. COVID appears to be here to stay, and I expect post-COVID syndrome is, too. A doctor is better able to assess how you are affected by COVID if you had a baseline assessment from before the injury, just like with concussions. Find a doctor trained in applied clinical neuroscience, a.k.a. functional neurology, and get baseline testing while you are healthy. Then, if you suffer from a concussion, COVID, or any other condition that compromises brain function, your doctor will be better able to see which areas are most affected and to recommend a treatment plan to help you regain your quality of life. If you have not already had baseline testing but suspect you are suffering from long COVID, find a doctor who can help. Sometimes, it's simply a matter of retraining the brain.

Dr. Marc Ellis is the clinic director at Georgia Chiropractic Neurology Center. By combining myofascial techniques with chiropractic and brain rehabilitation to address the patient in an integrated manner, Dr. Ellis presents a rare combination of healing skills that reflect an inborn talent to restore proper function to the human body. He is a founding member of the International Fascial Research Congress. He was valedictorian of the Carrick Institute in 2004 and went on to become an assistant professor of neurology for the Carrick Institute. He also developed his own technique called MyoSynaptics, which integrates manual therapy with brain rehab. Dr. Ellis is published in peer-reviewed journals and has over 20 years of teaching experience.

Chapter 7

How Yoga Helped Me Rehab My
Traumatic Brain Injury

By Amy Zellmer

On a cold February morning, my life changed for-ever. Walking down the driveway of my building, I slipped on a patch of sheer ice. My feet went straight up, and when I landed, my head took the full impact, briefly knocking me unconscious.

As I started to get up, I knew I wasn't okay. I had an excruciating pain in my skull where it hit, and I was seeing whirly, bright lights out of my left eye.

The doctor confirmed I had a severe concussion, major whiplash, C4/5 damage, a dislocated sternum, and multiple torn muscles. I had no idea the road to recovery I'd face — nor how drastically my life had just changed.

I had been doing yoga since college because it brought me balance and peace and was an instant de-stressor me. With all of my physical injuries due to my traumatic brain injury (TBI), I could no longer do yoga.

After months of vertigo, dizziness, balance issues, cognitive problems, short-term memory loss, and the pain of my physical injuries, I was at the end of my rope. I felt like

I would never find any relief and worried that the TBI would leave me permanently impaired and unable to ever do physical exercise again.

I consulted with a neurologist, a chiropractic neurologist, as well as the National Balance and Dizzy Center. I was encouraged to attempt some physical movement, as it would eventually help my body work out its kinks and stabilize my balance issues. It seemed counterintuitive at the time; however, I was desperate to have some sense of normalcy and routine in my life.

About fifteen months after my accident, I took private lessons with my yoga instructor in an attempt to find poses I could do — poses that wouldn't trigger my vertigo or cause tension in my neck or sternum/clavicle area.

My instructor taught me how to use a chair or wall to support myself in standing poses so I didn't feel like I was going to fall. We found five poses I could do with modifications that didn't cause any problems or flare-ups: Tree, Mountain, Cat/Cow, Puppy Dog, Forward Bend, and Seated Spine Twist.

Within about six weeks of doing these five poses every day for 10 minutes, I gradually added Down Dog, Plank, and Warrior for one breath each. My vertigo and dizzy issues seemed to almost completely subside, and my balance was coming back, closer to what it was pre-accident. Now, with modifications, I can do many of the poses I used to do. I still can't do any back bends or tip my head backwards, but I am on an amazing road to recovery, thanks to yoga.

I urge anyone with a TBI or other injury to try to incorporate yoga into your daily routine. If you think, "I'm not flexible, I can't do yoga," be kind to yourself and try it slowly! If I can do this, I know you can too.

A few tips as you begin your yoga practice:

1. Listen to your body. Don't do anything that hurts or causes you pain. Mild discomfort is to be expected if you haven't stretched your body in a while; however, if it actually hurts, listen to your body. Don't do that particular pose, or modify it to fit what your body is capable of. If a pose triggers vertigo, try modifying it so that your head doesn't have to move, or else move on to a different pose.

2. Connect your breath. Oxygen is critical for brain health, and yoga helps you connect your breath to your movements. Take strong, deep inhalations, and allow the out-breath to help you get deeper into the pose and deeper into the now, releasing all negative thoughts and emotions.

3. Modify poses. In the beginning, I could only do five simple, basic, stretching poses. I had to use a chair or wall to hold onto for balance. I couldn't do any poses that required my head to be forward or backward. Don't feel obligated to do every pose in a series; do what you can do and go at your own pace. Yoga is an individual "sport," and there is no one to impress.

4. Find an instructor knowledgeable about accessible yoga and disabilities who can help you create an individualized flow that is doable from the comfort of your own home. It's not about doing a big pose; it's about getting movement and breath into your body — even if you practice seated in a chair.

5. Believe in yourself. I know it's a challenge when you haven't been able to do physical exercise in months, but I finally took the plunge, and I know you can too! Yoga has so many health benefits, and I truly believe in you and your ability to get moving and start feeling better. Let go of the resistance that is holding you back, and allow yourself to move forward in your recovery. Your mind, body, and spirit will thank you!

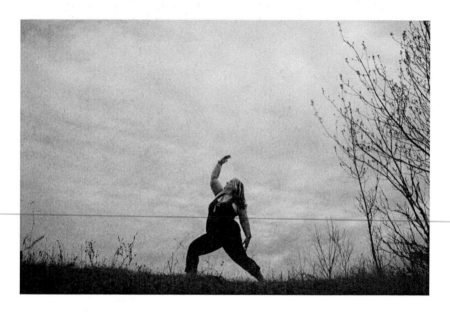

Brain-Boosting Yoga

Have you heard the saying, "Neurons that fire together, wire together?"

Okay, maybe I'm the only neuro-geek in the room, but that is exactly what we are doing in a brain-boosting yoga practice. When neurons wire together, neuroplasticity happens, which is our brain's ability to adapt and create new pathways. It's especially important for anyone in cognitive decline.

Did you know that after the age of approximately 25, our brain begins declining? So when I say "anyone in cognitive decline," I am referring to anyone in their late 20s and up. *Everyone* needs to be concerned about their brain health, no matter their age, because if your brain isn't developing, it's declining. But we can slow down the decline with neuroplasticity!

Forcing the left and right hemispheres to work together in brain-boosting yoga, while purposefully confusing the brain and challenging it to learn new information, is exactly what we need in order to keep our brains firing on all cylinders, and it's exactly how neuroplasticity happens.

Yoga in general will help you feel more at ease and begin to have more endurance. When we focus specifically on brain-boosting yoga, we can create changes in our brains — and in our bodies and lives.

Strategically using contralateral, cross-lateral, midline, and gaze stability exercises in conjunction with "resetting" poses (such as gentle forward folds) and breathwork, we give our brains important neurological information:

1. proprioception (where we are in space)
2. visual-spatial awareness (depth perception)
3. vestibular input (sensations of the movement of the head or body)
4. parasympathetic activation ("rest and digest" mode)

5. improved tone of the vagal nerve
6. nervous system resilience

Every *body* really can do yoga, regardless of size, flexibility, ability, and injury. My brain-boosting yoga style is slow, gentle, and intentional. If you have balance or mobility issues, you can get the same benefits by doing the practice seated in a chair. The key is consistency; you can't just try it once and say whether it worked or not. You need to consistently practice 3-5 times a week to give the brain a chance to develop neuroplasticity and create lasting changes.

Conclusion

There are plenty of other benefits of yoga, including improved flexibility, increased strength, better balance, more restful sleep, improved relationships (like less fighting because you are less stressed), enhanced mobility, calming of the sympathetic nervous system (getting you out of fight-or-flight mode), and improved gut function.

My own experience motivated me to help others experience the power of yoga in their own recovery, whether it's from a TBI or a different injury or illness — or even if they are just looking for a way to de-stress in their busy lives.

Whatever your reason for coming to yoga, I am passionate about helping you realize your full potential and helping you get better tuned in to your body. Many will not need modifications, but for those who do, I am confident that you will still get plenty of benefits from a regular practice.

Amy Zellmer is a TBI survivor and award-winning author of Life With a Traumatic Brain Injury: Finding the Road Back to Normal. She is the founder and editor-in-chief of The Brain Health Magazine as well as a national speaker and leader in the movement for TBI awareness. She hosts the number-one podcast for concussion and TBI resources, "Faces of TBI." She is also editor-in-chief of MN YOGA + Life Magazine and has a passion to spread the message that yoga is for every body, regardless of size or ability. She is a registered yoga instructor, having completed 200 hours of teacher training, and she is in the process of completing her 500-hour teacher training. She is also certified in trauma-informed yoga, LoveYourBrain yoga, chair yoga, and the body-positive Yoga For All. Additionally, she hosts a podcast series, "Creating Wellness From Within." Join Amy on Patreon for weekly brain-boosting yoga classes via Zoom: www.patreon.com/amyzellmer.

Chapter 8

Improving Neurological Blood Flow with Acupuncture

By Dr. Clayton Shiu, PhD

I founded the Shiu Clinic to offer patients a combination of traditional Chinese medicine and neuroscience-based acupuncture with Western medicine, in a pioneering program that includes the use of innovative, cutting-edge technology and techniques. This approach is achieving unparalleled results for concussion patients experiencing a host of symptoms.

I completed my doctoral studies at the premier stroke and neurological hospital in China under its founder, Dr. Shi Xue Min, who is known as the father of modern acupuncture and stroke therapy. He conducted groundbreaking research that determined which acupuncture points can increase blood flow to the brain, and through him, I learned how to manipulate brain blood flow.

Subsequently, I developed a neurological acupuncture treatment system — Nanopuncture® and Neural Flush — that allows me to analyze where a patient's circulation is inhibited and to directly reset and reboot the nervous system to increase neuromuscular circulation.

Every cell in the central nervous system needs constant blood flow, and any loss of blood flow, no matter how brief, is considered a stroke. Strokes can be caused by internal, constitutional causes or by external factors such as traumatic brain injury (TBI) or concussion.

The Nanopuncture® and Neural Flush systems integrate Western neurological analysis and Eastern medicine knowledge of the tendinomuscular meridians of the body, restoring healthy blood flow to the brain and spinal cord and allowing nerves to reawaken and regenerate.

At the Shiu Clinic, we specialize in treating cerebral and neurological disorders — including stroke, Parkinson's, paralysis, and TBIs such as concussions — using our Awakening program, a treatment plan that is customized for individual patients. It incorporates acupuncture, neurofeedback with advanced technology real-time brain mapping, assessment and treatment of the neck to insure healthy blood flow, and photobiomodulation (PBM) light therapy to reduce inflammation, as well as traditional Chinese herbal medicine and other modalities such as physical therapy, massage, and nutritional counseling.

Shiu Clinic practitioners in different areas of specialization work seamlessly as a team to care for each of our patients. During our TBI patient's initial visit to the clinic, the team gathers to meet the patient and analyze their imaging, bloodwork, and other medical data from prior to the TBI event. It's important that we take a thorough history, much like reconstructing a detective story. Often, it's not just an event or accident that created the injury — prior medical history can play a role.

We take a multi-pronged approach:

1. We use traditional Chinese medicine diagnostic tools, such as assessing the pulses and examining the tongue. This provides additional information to inform the development of a treatment plan.
2. As part of the Nanopuncture® system, we use specific methods to palpate and treat meridians along the neck and skull.
3. We conduct standard neurological testing to assess which lobes of the brain are affected by the traumatic injury.
4. In addition, we highly recommend that the patient undergo a qEEG (Qualitative Electrocncephalogram) brain scan, which is done right on site with our qEEG specialist, Dr. Valentina Duque.

The Nanopuncture® approach to treating concussions includes a specific methodology for assessing the neck, which acts as a natural shock absorber whenever a concussion occurs. In its efforts to protect and stabilize the head, the neck also, unfortunately, retains trapped inflammation, which impacts major superhighway blood vessels like the vertebral basilar artery and the paraspinal arteries. This, in turn, affects the circle of Willis, which is a huge network of blood vessels, and impacts the supply of oxygenated blood to the brain.

The qEEG measures electrical activity in the form of brain wave patterns (sometimes referred to as "brain mapping"). The qEEG Brainmaster technology gives us a live, real-time, computer-generated image of the TBI patient's brain and its health, providing baseline data about brain function and circulation as well as insight into whether the patient is under- or over-medicated or has a severe history of concussion, dyslexia, or ADHD, or if the overall brain wave activities are unbalanced.

The live scan informs our decisions about acupuncture treatment, focusing on particular parts of the brain as well as our development of a neurofeedback training program to help the patient retrain their brain and reduce abnormal brain activity.

Also, we are fortunate at the Shiu Clinic to have the use of highly efficacious new PBM devices that use different wavelengths and pulsing frequencies of light to interact with the cells in our body, increasing circulation, reducing inflammation, and decreasing fatigue. We have developed a relationship with the Vielight company, and over the years, we have researched and used their PBM headset devices to treat the brainwaves of TBI patients. These treatments can directly target injured brain cells, accelerating neurological repair and improving the function of the systems regulating cognitive function, attention, memory, emotions, and behavior.

In addition to using handheld light devices, we are one of the few clinics in the United States to employ a full-body ReGen Pod, which provides 360-degree, high-intensity, LED-technology laser light treatment. The Shiu Clinic staff is very experienced in the use of the ReGen Pod machines, and we have developed different customized pulse and wavelength frequencies for each of our TBI patients to achieve best results.

Case Study: Treating Zoe with the Awakening Program

Zoe was referred to our clinic by her other doctors. Many of the concussion patients we meet are, understandably, very concerned about their injuries and anxious about the possibility of getting re-injured, and Zoe was hesitant when entering the office.

Unfortunately, Zoe had suffered multiple concussions, which continued to spiral into migraine headache symptoms. Her first concussion had been four years earlier — ironically, while she was a medical student studying neuroscience. The concussion was initiated by metal headphones that suddenly folded up and hit the back of the mastoid bones of her head. Like many concussion victims, she ignored the impact and continued going about her day, including attending a kickboxing class, which continued to enrage the concussion. Her head injury worsened, manifesting symptoms of dizziness, and she took a month off from medical school.

As her symptoms worsened, she also began to have gait issues. Later that year, she fell down the stairs, suffering another impact, and subsequently took a full year off from school. Her symptoms continued to increase.

In addition to migraine headaches, her eyes became very sensitive to light, and she was unable to work on the computer. She had previously tried acupuncture, but discontinued it because she found it painful, without bringing much relief.

The following year, she was dancing at home, in her socks, and slipped and fell on the right side of her head, simultaneously damaging her hip bones. She then started to exhibit dysautonomia symptoms such as extreme nausea, panic attacks, unusual spontaneous sweating, ringing in the ears, pain behind the eyes, insomnia, and partial orthostatic hypertension.

At this point, she was so sensitive that even gently touching the table she was lying on would trigger a severe response. Her body was sensitive to the lights and sounds in the treatment room, so we turned the lights off and lowered the music until it was barely audible.

Despite the cumulative impacts of Zoe's repeated injuries, we were able to clear up all of her symptoms, allowing her to resume her normal life and return to school. It took time, but the key factors, which are unique to our approach, were our detailed examination of her neck and the development of a custom treatment plan that increased healthy blood flow.

Upon first visual examination and palpation of her neck, we noticed an enormous amount of stiffness and inflammation. The swelling was disrupting the vertebral basilar artery, which supplies blood to the circle of Willis and thus many neural structures in the skull. There was damage to the vagus nerve, which controls bodily functions such as digestion, heart rate, and the immune system. Zoe was also experiencing lightheadedness and a loss of balance. A full neurological examination revealed that her brain's frontal lobe, parietal lobe, and cerebellum were affected.

In these kinds of cases, we position the patient on their side, in the fetal position, and place acupuncture needles behind the head and neck to start restoring the body's natural spring and shock absorber.

Then, I palpated her stomach and found an intense pounding in her belly from the abdominal aorta, which indicated a hyperactive sympathetic nervous system. Digestive issues, which Zoe had experienced prior to her injuries, were getting worse, exacerbated by her TBI. Because of these digestive symptoms, we booked a thorough herbal consultation with our Herbal Director, Jeffrey Chen.

Also, to reduce fatigue and energize her body, we had Zoe undergo a full light treatment in the ReGen Pod twice a week during the first month of treatment.

Zoe's progress was tracked and her treatment plan re-evaluated regularly after a series of 10 treatments, which is considered the minimum necessary to produce neuroplasticity changes.

After about two months of her Awakening program treatment, Zoe's symptoms had improved by about 85 percent. As the inflammation in her neck abated, she was able to better focus her eyes, allowing her to do computer work. She also became less sensitive to light. Her body started to feel much more resilient, and she returned to the gym, working out on machines and doing cardio. In addition, her customized herbal medicine formula soothed her sympathetic nervous system, so her poor digestion, diarrhea, and constipation subsided completely.

Conclusion

Once our Shiu Clinic patients have progressed through the various elements of their Awakening program, which may occur over a course of two weeks to several months, a follow-up brain scan is performed to get objective data on their progress and to guide our staff in adjusting the program. Aftercare can include the use of recommended at-home PBM, neurofeedback, or other machines as well as ongoing herbal medicine assessments and nutritional guidance.

Through the holistic and seamless integration of the full range of powerful healing tools at our disposal — both ancient and modern — concussion patients can awaken once again to good health.

Dr. Clayton Shiu is at the forefront of integrating acupuncture with Western medicine for optimal patient care and powerful outcomes. Dr. Shiu earned a Bachelor of Science in Human Physiology from Boston University, a Master of Science in Traditional Oriental Medicine from Pacific College of Oriental Medicine, and a PhD in Acupuncture and Moxibustion from the Tianjin University of Traditional Chinese Medicine. He completed his residency at the First Teaching Hospital of Tianjin (which is featured in the acclaimed documentary *9,000 Needles*) and continued to refine his understanding of Chinese medicine under many renowned teachers, most notably Dr. Shi Xue Min, a stroke specialist and the father of modern acupuncture.

Dr. Shiu *is the creator of the stroke and neurological rehabilitation system Nanopuncture®, which he teaches to acupuncturists and other medical professionals across the country. In 2019, he founded The Shiu Clinic, the first in New York City to combine neuroscience, acupuncture, and the most cutting-edge PBM technology. Dr. Shiu holds faculty positions at the Academy of Chinese Culture and Health Sciences and the American College of Traditional Chinese Medicine, teaching stroke rehabilitation courses for their doctoral programs. He has been featured in Reuters and in two recently published books: Creative Success Now: How Creatives Can Thrive in the 21st Century and Fix My Face: Expert Advice for Maximizing Recovery from Bell's Palsy, Ramsay Hunt Syndrome, and Other Causes of Facial Nerve Paralysis.*

Chapter 9

The Risk of Dementia after TBI
By Dr. Eric Kaplan, DC, DACNB, FACFN, FABVR, FABCDD

In the United States, 1.7 million individuals are estimated to sustain a traumatic brain injury (TBI) annually.[9] There are different types of TBIs, but falls are the leading cause. Adults who are 75 years or older have the highest percent of having a hospitalization or death resulting from a fall,[10] so vestibular rehabilitation focused on fall prevention can be vital to ensuring a high quality of life for senior citizens. After falls, the next two most common causes of TBIs are car accidents and sports injuries. People also have severe head injuries from shockwaves in battlefields, bullets hitting the head, work accidents, and, unfortunately, domestic violence.

---

[9] Langlois JA, Rutland-Brown W, Thomas KE. Traumatic brain injury in the United States; emergency department visits, hospitalizations, and deaths. National Center for Injury Prevention and Control (U.S.), Division of Injury Response. 2006 Jan [cited 9 Aug 2022]. Available from: https://stacks.cdc.gov/view/cdc/12294.

[10] Schwenkreis P, Gonschorek A, Berg F, Meier U, Rogge W, Schmehl I, et al. Prospective observational cohort study on epidemiology, treatment and outcome of patients with traumatic brain injury (TBI) in German BG hospitals. BMJ Open. 2021 Jun 4;11(6):e045771. doi: 10.1136/bmjopen-2020-045771. PMID: 34088707; PMCID: PMC8183205.

TBIs can result in losing consciousness, forgetfulness, temporary amnesia, confusion, visual disturbances, headaches, dizziness, seizures, light and sound sensitivity, trouble with focus, memory loss, trouble with walking, trouble with talking, and many more problems. Researchers have also come to the conclusion that if the head injury is very severe, it can even lead to neurological disorders such as Alzheimer's disease (AD). In fact, one of the most researched topics in AD is TBI.

AD is one of the fastest-growing health conditions. From 1999 to 2019, the U.S. mortality rate from AD in the overall population significantly increased from 16 to 30 deaths per 100,000, an 88% increase.[11] Prevalence/incidence studies reported at the 2021 Alzheimer's Association International Conference, the world's largest conference for dementia research, found that each year, an estimated 10 in every 100,000 individuals develop dementia with early onset (prior to age 65).[12] This corresponds to 350,000 new cases of early onset dementia per year, globally. Because of these significant numbers, we need to find out the reasons why these numbers are increasing as well as ways to stop the progression and prevent dementia or Alzheimers from developing in the first place.

However, one of the problems with researching AD is that scientists often have to rely on the autopsy at death to

---

[11] Nordström A, Nordström P. Traumatic brain injury and the risk of dementia diagnosis: A nationwide cohort study. PLoS Med. 2018 Jan 30;15(1):e1002496. doi: 10.1371/journal.pmed.1002496. PMID: 29381704; PMCID: PMC5790223.

[12] Hendriks S, Peetoom K, Bakker C, van der Flier WM, Papma JM, Koopmans R, et al. Global Prevalence of Young-Onset Dementia: A Systematic Review and Meta-analysis. JAMA Neurol. 2021 Sep 1;78(9):1080-1090. doi: 10.1001/jamaneurol.2021.2161. PMID: 34279544; PMCID: PMC8290331.

really determine how AD affected the brain. During an autopsy, scientists look for tau proteins and amyloid plaques. These tau proteins form abnormally and cling to other tau proteins to form so-called "tau tangles" inside the brain cells. Tau tangles and beta-amyloid plaques are large accumulations of microscopic brain protein fragments that slow a person's ability to think and remember, and they are very apparent in AD.

In addition to the upregulation of beta-amyloid protein precursors, it has been hypothesized that the presence of plaques following a TBI may be due to damaged axons that contribute to amyloid protein accumulation.[13] These axons are nerve fibers that help connect different cells in the brain, but when damaged in a TBI, they may be the site of amyloid protein accumulation.

A Finnish study showed that there is a greater chance of developing dementia later on in life if you have had a severe TBI as opposed to a mild TBI[11]. Interestingly, the study also found that people with multiple TBIs or more severe TBIs did have lower cognitive function even before their head injuries.[14]

Although the research with mild traumatic brain injuries has been inconclusive, if there is a major or severe head injury with loss of consciousness, especially if it lasts

[13] Smith DH, Chen XH, Iwata A, Graham DI. Amyloid beta accumulation in axons after traumatic brain injury in humans. J Neurosurg. 2003 May;98(5):1072-7. doi: 10.3171/jns.2003.98.5.1072. PMID: 12744368.
[14] Raj R, Kaprio J, Jousilahti P, Korja M, Siironen J. Risk of Dementia After Hospitalization Due to Traumatic Brain Injury: A Longitudinal, Population-Based Study. Neurology. 2022 May 11:10.1212/WNL.0000000000200290. doi: 10.1212/WNL.0000000000200290. Epub ahead of print. PMID: 35545443.

more than five minutes, the person is likely to be diagnosed with dementia within the first year, and it may even lead to AD years later.[15] The more severe the injury, the greater the chance of a poor outcome.

Not only are the outcomes worse if the TBI is severe, but they are also worse if you have had multiple head injuries that result in what is called chronic traumatic encephalopathy (CTE). In football or hockey for example, the player's heads are hit over and over again. Many players unknowingly cause their own injuries by hitting an opponent with their head first and even purposely banging teammates' helmets together in celebration.

Unfortunately, some players believe that the helmet is protecting their brains from concussion, but the truth is they can still get a concussion caused by diffuse axonal injury, internal shearing forces, coup-contrecoup injuries, and even abnormal torquing. Additionally, the head injuries are not always at the point of impact, and although the risk of brain dysfunction or dementia is highest after the first year of a head injury, research has shown damage can be sustained 30 years later.[14]

In another recent study, the risk of a dementia diagnosis was increased by about 80% during an average follow-up period of 15 years for individuals diagnosed with TBI.[11] The study also found that the risk of being diagnosed with dementia in the first year after TBI was four to six times higher when compared with individuals with no TBI.[11] The

[15] Fernández-Blázquez MA, Noriega-Ruiz B, Ávila-Villanueva M, Valentí-Soler M, Frades-Payo B, Del Ser T, Gómez-Ramírez J. Impact of individual and neighborhood dimensions of socioeconomic status on the prevalence of mild cognitive impairment over seven-year follow-up. Aging Ment Health. 2021 May;25(5):814-823. doi: 10.1080/13607863.2020.1725803. Epub 2020 Feb 18. PMID: 32067489.

development of dementia, with impaired executive function, an increased risk of falling, and reduced cognitive function was significantly associated and observed more than 30 years after TBI.

What this means is that your past head injury can cause problems later in life, so it is best to take care of any dysfunction now, before it progresses. If you have had any type of head injury, whether it is from playing sports, a car accident, or a slip and fall, it is vital to get your brain analyzed with a full neurological evaluation to figure out what areas, if any, are not functioning at optimal levels. Therefore, you can improve your brain function now and prevent future neurological problems such as dementia, AD, or Parkinson's disease.

Do not wait until you get one of these severe neurological disorders to start working on your health because there are usually early clues or signs that the brain is not working properly. For example, someone might complain of brain fog, trouble with focus, low energy, headaches, dizziness, visual disturbances, poor memory, decreased motivation, depression, or anxiety, and might not realize that their neurological problems may be related to an accident or head injury. These are early warning signs that you need to get a neurological examination to determine if there is any risk for dementia or AD.

Be sure to share information with your doctor that might be significant, such as any past history of physical or emotional trauma, sports injuries, slips and falls, chemical exposures, car accidents, physical altercations, and even problems with pregnancy and infancy. The more symptoms of mild dementia or early-stage AD, the greater the chance of progression. For example, diminished short-term memory, misplacing belongings in odd places, and difficulty finding the right name or word are the most common complaints and signs of early onset AD. A lot of times, people also state that since their TBI, they do not seem like themselves. They may have lapses in judgment, have difficulty with mental arithmetic, show uncharacteristic behaviors, and have trouble handling money. Disorientation in unfamiliar places or situations is also an early sign of dementia, as well as becoming more apathetic or withdrawn, such as avoiding social situations. Lastly, other significant complaints with dementia or early onset AD are difficulty with routine tasks at work or at home, taking longer to complete tasks, and irritation or anger in response to increasing memory lapses.

One test that is commonly used to determine if there is such a risk is called the MoCA (Montreal Cognitive Assessment) Test for Dementia. It is a very simple and brief test that is a reliable screening tool for AD. It checks executive functions, orientation, memory, visual spatial ability, language, math, recall, and abstraction. It is only 30 questions and takes about 10 minutes to complete. A normal score is 26 or above out of possible 30. If the score is less than 26, it is considered abnormal and would require further intervention. A follow-up test using different questions should be taken after treatment is performed to see if there is improvement in the MoCA Test for Dementia.

Most likely, there is also a relationship with dementia and a person's upbringing,[15] education,[16] and genetics. Regarding the latter, you may be wondering: Is there anything you can do on your own to help yourself prevent future problems, or do your genes dictate your future?

When answering questions about genetics, it is always good to look at siblings because they have the most similar genes. One research study compared 47,000 full sibling pairs and found that if one sibling has had a TBI, they are twice as likely to develop dementia than the other sibling who has not had a TBI.[11] They followed up with these siblings 10 years later to find that the increase in dementia remained the same after all of those years as well. Based on this, it is highly likely that the environment can alter brain function as well as gene expression.

The bad news is that head injuries can cause future brain problems, but the good news is that you can also alter environmental factors to help with current brain problems and prevent future brain problems. One environmental factor is a healthy diet or having the proper nutritional program.

There has been research in support of taking neuroprotective nutrients because they can alter gene expression and have a positive effect on health and prevention of neurodegenerative disorders. What this means is that by altering your diet, you can help prevent dysfunction of the

---

[16] Takasugi T, Tsuji T, Hanazato M, Miyaguni Y, Ojima T, Kondo K. Community-level educational attainment and dementia: a 6-year longitudinal multilevel study in Japan. BMC Geriatr. 2021 Nov 23;21(1):661. doi: 10.1186/s12877-021-02615-x. Erratum in: BMC Geriatr. 2021 Dec 15;21(1):709. PMID: 34814847; PMCID: PMC8609807.

brain and nervous system. Folate, B12, choline, zinc, selenium, and dietary polyphenols are capable of interacting with epigenetic mechanisms and ultimately gene expression[17]. Since epigenetic mechanisms resulting in neuronal dysfunction are ultimately affected by diet, with certain nutritional protocols or programs, we can decrease the vulnerability of neurons to degeneration which is seen in AD.

Another factor to consider after a head injury is that a vitamin D deficiency may increase your risk of A.[18] Therefore, if you have had a concussion or traumatic brain injury, it is important to analyze blood work for the appropriate vitamin D levels, which should be at least 35 ng/mL. One way to increase these levels is to go outside for 20 minutes between 12 p.m. and 2 p.m. when the sun is strongest and absorption will be greatest. If you have a history of skin cancer or sunburn, the healthiest way to protect yourself is to use zinc oxide on areas of the skin that are exposed the most. Additionally, salmon, eggs, cod liver oil, and sardines are good dietary sources of vitamin D. Vitamin D supplements can also be useful but must be taken with fat and vitamin K for best absorption.

Intermittent fasting and getting proper sleep can also help prevent AD and deposition of beta-amyloid plaques.[19]

[17] Sezgin Z, Dincer Y. Alzheimer's disease and epigenetic diet. Neurochem Int. 2014 Dec;78:105-16. doi: 10.1016/j.neuint.2014.09.012. Epub 2014 Oct 5. PMID: 25290336.

[18] Lu'o'ng KV, Nguyên LT. The beneficial role of vitamin D in Alzheimer's disease. Am J Alzheimers Dis Other Demen. 2011 Nov;26(7):511-20. doi: 10.1177/1533317511429321. Epub 2011 Dec 27. PMID: 22202127.

[19] Zhang J, Zhan Z, Li X, Xing A, Jiang C, Chen Y, Shi W, An L. Intermittent fasting protects against Alzheimer's Disease possible through restoring aquaporin-4 polarity. Front Mol Neurosci. 2017 Nov 29;10:395. doi: 10.3389/fnmol.2017.00395. PMID: 29238290; PMCID: PMC5712566.

Intermittent fasting is when you eat only eight hours a day and fast for 16 hours a day. For example, if you eat from 10 a.m. to 6 p.m. and sleep from 10 p.m. to 6 a.m., you have a better chance of improving brain function than if you were eating all day and not sleeping properly.

In addition to monitoring eating and sleeping habits, it is also important to analyze your blood work. Recently, there has been a lot of talk and studies linking diabetes to AD. Researchers are even contemplating changing the name of AD to Diabetes Type 3.[20] Therefore, if you have had a TBI, it is important to maintain healthy glucose levels.

When getting blood work done, it is best if your fasting blood glucose is less than 100 mg/dL to ensure proper brain function. Also, check your Hemoglobin AIC, which is the main test to help you manage your diabetes. Hemoglobin AIC is measuring your average blood glucose over the previous three months. The ideal range would be under 5.7%. People whose Hemoglobin AIC is above 5.7% and who have a fasting glucose of more than 100 mg/dL may complain of increased thirst, increased urination, blurred vision, fatigue, and even nerve pain. If you have had some of these symptoms and your blood work glucose numbers are high and you have a history of concussions, your chances of developing AD and dementia are greatly increased. The next step is to improve your diabetes numbers with diet and exercise, as well as to get help with any areas of the brain that were injured during the concussion.

---

[20] Nguyen TT, Ta QTH, Nguyen TKO, Nguyen TTD, Giau VV. Type 3 diabetes and its role implications in Alzheimer's Disease. Int J Mol Sci. 2020 Apr 30;21(9):3165. doi: 10.3390/ijms21093165. PMID: 32365816; PMCID: PMC7246646.

So even though the research shows that you are more likely to develop dementia or AD if you had a severe TBI, there are many intrinsic stimuli and environmental factors that you can change to decrease your chances of degenerative neurological disorders. Do not wait until the symptoms get worse before you do something about it. If you have ever had a traumatic brain injury or concussion, it is important to make progress in your health, work on factors that you can control, monitor your biomarkers to ensure your interventions are working correctly, and get to the root of your TBI symptoms to improve your quality of life and prevent future neurological disorders such as AD.

Dr. Eric Kaplan is an open, eager, enthusiastic teacher and student of the world of health and wellness. Dr. Kaplan received a B.S. in Human Biology at Emory University and a D.C. from Palmer College of Chiropractic-West. In addition, he is a board-certified functional neurologist with over 1,500 hours of post-graduate studies at The Carrick Institute, including specialty courses such as Traumatic Brain Injury (TBI), Movement Disorders, and Coma. He also completed three fellowships through the American College of Functional Neurology, the American Board of Vestibular Rehabilitation, and the American Board of Childhood Developmental Delays. Being trained in dozens of functional and neurological techniques, he has the ability to treat many different types of patients.

Dr. Kaplan is also the founder and sole proprietor of Kaplan Brain & Body, two full-service functional neurology and functional medicine wellness centers located in the heart of the West Village in New York City and in Bergen County, New Jersey. Having served patients for over 22 years, Dr. Kaplan is committed not only to his patients' health but to the overall quality of their lives. The Kaplan Brain & Body philosophy integrates the physical wellness side of life with the human side. Any Kaplan Brain & Body patient will tell you Dr. Kaplan is a warm, passionate, and inspirational teacher of love, health, and happiness. He also was the head neurology professor at TriSate College in Manhattan, is currently the health columnist for the Pascack Press in Bergen County, NJ, and radio host of Boost Your Brain Power with Dr. Eric Kaplan on AM 970, and is author of Boost Your Brain Power: A Guide to Improving Your Memory and Focus

Chapter 10

The Link between Brain Injury and Dementia
By Dr. Kassie Kaas

"Don't deny the diagnosis, defy the verdict."
– Dr. Norman Cousins, *Anatomy of an Illness*

The Brain Injury Alliance of America estimates that more than 3.5 million brain injuries occur each year. This translates to a brain injury being sustained by someone in the U.S. every nine seconds. Mild traumatic brain injuries (mTBI), also referred to as concussions, do not necessarily involve a loss of consciousness, but often lead to symptoms that can linger for weeks, months, or longer. All traumatic brain injuries (TBI) can carry health consequences that continue long after the impact. All too often, these consequences will go overlooked and be dismissed by healthcare professionals, especially in instances where the patient "looks fine." Physical trauma can happen to the brain while leaving little visible evidence on traditional imaging and scans such as an MRI or CT. These "invisible injuries" can have significant influence on future brain health status and the development of dementia.

This connection leads to an important question: Does sustaining a brain injury always increase the likelihood of developing dementia later in life, and can anything be done to prevent or reverse the neurodegenerative process?

"Dementia" is an overall term for a particular group of symptoms, often including memory deficits, visual-spatial and language issues, emotional or personality changes, and problem-solving difficulties. Dementia becomes more common as we age, but it is not a normal part of the aging process.

Alzheimer's disease (AD) is one of the most predominant causes of dementia. An estimated 6.5 million Americans age 65 and older are living with AD in 2022, according to the Alzheimer's Association. AD affects approximately one out of nine individuals age 65 and older.

Both TBI and AD impact a significant number of people. By studying the pathological changes that occur in a TBI, it could become possible to identify key pathways and neurometabolic processes that lead to further neurodegeneration, allowing us a way to potentially address the decline, slowing, or stopping of its progression during the normal course of aging.

According to the Alzheimer's Association, key studies have shown that older adults with a history of moderate TBI are 2.3 times more likely to develop AD than seniors with no history of head injury, and those with a history of severe TBI are 4.5 times more likely to develop AD. There is no clear evidence to show that a single mTBI increases dementia risk; however, research does indicate that repeated mild brain injuries may be linked to the neurodegenerative disorder Chronic Traumatic Encephalopathy

(CTE). Additionally, a history of TBI may accelerate the onset of cognitive impairment by two or more years, making sustaining a TBI a significant risk factor for early cognitive decline.

Brain mapping studies have identified substantial similarities in the neurodegenerative patterns associated with AD and mTBI. Brain injuries of all kinds are often followed by a series of persistent aftereffects including headaches, issues with word finding, decision-making difficulties, inability to focus, changes in balance, reduced neural processing speed, and memory deficits. Many of these same symptoms are hallmarks of AD and other dementias.

A study published in 2021 demonstrated that there were similar identifiable changes in the brains of people who had mTBI and those diagnosed with AD. The researchers showed that there was a reduction in cortical thickness of the brain and parallel patterns of cerebral white matter degradation as compared to uninjured brains. The study also investigated outcomes of sustaining a mTBI later in life and found geriatric mTBI patients to be significantly more likely than typically aging adults to exhibit AD-like trajectories of neurodegeneration, even as early as six months post-injury.[21]

Researchers have studied many neural mechanisms that result in age-related dementias like AD, such as brain volume changes, atrophy in specific areas, and lack of nu-

[21] Rostowsky KA, Irimia A; Alzheimer's Disease Neuroimaging Initiative. Acute cognitive impairment after traumatic brain injury predicts the occurrence of brain atrophy patterns similar to those observed in Alzheimer's disease. Geroscience. 2021 Aug;43(4):2015-2039. doi: 10.1007/s11357-021-00355-9. Epub 2021 Apr 26. PMID: 33900530; PMCID: PMC8492819.

tritional support. Additionally, they have found that degeneration in the frontal and temporal lobes of the brain is associated with frontotemporal dementia, and destruction in the basal ganglia is related to the development of Parkinson's disease. Researchers have found protein tangles and plaques in the hippocampus of AD patients and build-ups of a protein called alpha-synuclein (termed "Lewy bodies") in the brain cells of the cerebral cortex, visual pathways, and brain stem in those with Lewy body dementia.

A toxic form of microtubule protein called Tau has been found in the brains of animal subjects post-TBI. It also plays a major pathological role in several types of dementia as well as CTE.

TBIs can trigger the formation of Tau build-ups, which can contribute to the development of tauopathy-related dementia, representing a link between TBI and dementia.

Many of the destructive metabolic processes and associated hallmark symptoms of these neurodegenerative diseases can overlap, so the term "mixed dementia" is often used. Symptoms observed and experienced often include poor memory, movement changes with walking or balance, development of a tremor, visual or auditory hallucinations, increased confusion, and changes in personality. These diseases are usually considered progressive, meaning the destruction keeps happening over time if not properly identified and addressed.

The traditional attitude surrounding cognitive decline is that nothing can be done to improve the symptoms or circumstances. Despite all of the ways one might develop some form of dementia, there is good news! The brain is capable of healing.

Numerous clinical trials, animal model studies, and published case study evidence have shown that with proper intervention, dysfunctional neural pathways can be overcome, and symptoms can improve. Neuroplasticity describes the brain's ability to change, modify, reorganize, and adjust in both function and structure in response to stimulus, activation, and experience. This is thrilling for those who have sustained a brain injury and/or are in cognitive decline.

The factors responsible for dysfunctional physiological pathways can be very different, so the modalities, care plans, therapies, and interventions applied should be just as unique as the individual and their history. The use of precision medicine and lifestyle modifications are the future of helping people overcome cognitive decline as well as brain injuries.

Over thirty years of medical investigation have put Dr. Dale Bredesen at the forefront of research into AD prevention and memory-loss reversal. His research teams have made discoveries that changed our understanding of the fundamental nature of AD and led to revolutionary treatments and a new lens through which to view the diagnosis of dementia.

Dr. Bredesen has outlined multiple (currently 36) factors that can trigger negative metabolic processes in the brain leading to cognitive decline and poor brain health. Comprehensive lab testing has been organized to help identify these factors on an individualized basis. Working with the results from the laboratory testing gives very detailed information on the potential drivers of the disease process and allows practitioners to address these factors and help their patients achieve better health outcomes.

Numerous studies and papers have been published showing how identifying and then optimizing these factors using distinct lifestyle modifications can slow cognitive decline processes and even reverse neurodegenerative symptoms. The Journal of Alzheimer's Disease recently published a clinical trial in which 25 patients diagnosed with dementia or mild cognitive impairment all showed statistically significant improvement in outcome measures after the application of a personalized, precision medicine approach.[22] Using the Bredesen Protocol made a measurable improvement in brain health.

One pertinent factor included in the Bredesen Protocol is a history of head trauma. The trauma may be mild and repetitive or more severe in nature. CTE is a well-studied consequence of head trauma and a tauopathy where disease progression can and often does continue in the absence of ongoing trauma. Commonly, a triad of aggression-depression-dementia symptomology is evident with this subset of the disease process.

These types of cases present themselves in the news with alarming frequency. Think of contact sport athletes who have been in the media for demonstrating out-of-character and dangerous behaviors, abusing substances,

---

[22] Toups K, Hathaway A, Gordon D, Chung H, Raji C, Boyd A, Hill BD, Hausman-Cohen S, Attarha M, Chwa WJ, Jarrett M, Bredesen DE. Precision Medicine Approach to Alzheimer's Disease: Successful Pilot Project. J Alzheimers Dis. 2022;88(4):1411-1421. doi: 10.3233/JAD-215707. PMID: 35811518.

committing acts of violence against their loved ones, succumbing to AD at a young age, or taking their own lives. These tragic circumstances could very well be the consequences of untreated head injuries that progressed into neurodegenerative disease patterns.

In the conventional model of care, very little is done to address this pathology. However, in a lifestyle and precision medicine approach like the Bredesen Protocol, positive action steps have been identified and well-studied.

Rehabilitation modalities such as hyperbaric oxygen therapy (HBOT) and exercise with oxygen therapy (EWOT) have been shown to improve cerebral blood flow. Low-level laser therapy (LLLT), sometimes referred to as cold laser or photobiomodulation (PBM), can help stabilize neurons, enhance mitochondrial output, and decrease inflammatory pathways in the brain. Optimizing nutrient and antioxidant levels such as vitamin D, magnesium, and glutathione can be beneficial in protecting brain health. Appropriate levels of hormones such as estrogen and progesterone, as well as the thyroid hormones, offer neuroprotection. Dietary supplements like vinpocetine and huperzine-A have been found to support blood flow and acetylcholine, the important neurotransmitter of learning and memory.

Increasing cardiovascular activity and health has demonstrated improved blood flow to the brain as well as increased production of important substances such as brain-derived neurotrophic factor (BDNF) and endorphins. BDNF is a vital protein that offers protection from neuroinflammation and supports neuronal survival while preventing cell death. Promoting pathways that upregulate BDNF, antioxidants, and key neurotransmitters will bring us so much farther in improving brain health and injury recovery than masking the symptoms.

Therapeutic modalities that address improving nutrition and supplementation support, exercise, sleep hygiene, stress support, cognitive stimulation, and optimizing our body's detoxification pathways have shown to increase neuroplasticity and positively transform cognitive performance. Whether or not a brain injury has been sustained, targeting and enhancing these key areas of health will only offer improved outcomes when it comes to brain function.

Unfortunately, drug trials aimed at addressing dementia and the AD epidemic have been a failure so far. Some offer minimal symptom relief, but none have offered any real hope of making lasting impacts on the neurodegenerative process. Fewer pharmaceuticals exist with the intent to improve the dysfunctional metabolism of an acquired brain injury, but there are numerous medications for managing the various symptoms that can persist after injury. However, these medications often produce other undesirable symptoms that may need to be managed over time. Healing can be a vicious cycle when interventions are not based on addressing the root cause of the dysfunction.

Strategies to increase or maintain cognitive health might help to prevent accelerated decline after sustaining a mTBI. An increased risk of dementia has been found in people with a history of TBI; however, a brain injury does not invariably lead to the development of dementia, and those diagnosed with dementia do not always have a history of brain injury. Regardless of the connection, it will always be well worth it to apply the principles of neuroplasticity for brain recovery and protection from future decline.

When you do not know better, you cannot do better. My mission is to help people understand that there are ways to support and optimize their brain health. No one has to sit back and accept decline as part of their health story. A brain injury does not have to lead to a dementia diagnosis, and a dementia diagnosis does not have to signify a rapid, irreversible decline in brain health. There is real hope in the fight against AD, and the time to start fighting is now.

Dr. Kassie Kaas earned her Bachelor of Science from the University of Minnesota-Duluth in biochemistry and molecular biology. She went on to earn her Doctorate of Chiropractic from Northwestern Health Sciences University. She has completed additional training in functional neurology and functional medicine. She also became a certified Bredesen Protocol practitioner so she could better serve patients diagnosed with cognitive decline, dementia and AD. Her primary focuses of care include brain injury rehabilitation, helping patients balance their hormones throughout life's transitions, and creating effective and comprehensive care plans for those suffering with cognitive decline, dementia, and AD. She is an active volunteer with the Alzheimer's Association and is passionate about educating people on how to protect and promote their brain health.

Chapter 11

Vestibular Concussions: A Case Review
By Dr. Cassandra Jimenez, DC, DACNB, FABVR and
Dr. Marc Ellis, DC, MSc, NMT, DACNB, FACFN, FABBIR

Functional neurologists understand that the brain is plastic, which means it can change no matter your age. We understand how to examine people and observe how their brain is functioning. We always keep in mind that each person's brain develops uniquely to them. Not only is each person's nervous system (of which the brain is a part) unique, but it functions differently on different days or at different times of the day. Some people have more energy in the morning while others have more later in the day.

As functional neurologists, we always pay attention to the individuality of the patient. While many of our treatment plans are similar, they are never quite the same. We would like to share the concussion story of someone who had a unique injury pattern that resulted in post-concussion syndrome with vertigo, headaches, and neck pain.

A Cycling Accident and Resulting Vertigo

James was a 65-year-old man who owned his own bicycle shop and was an avid cyclist until he had an accident in November of 2020. He fell while riding and hit his head, leaving him with post-concussion syndrome. James, like so many other people who suffer from concussions, saw numerous doctors until being referred to our office at the Georgia Chiropractic Neurology Center.

James came to our office about one year after his accident, complaining of vertigo, headaches, neck pain, loss of energy, depression, and insomnia. He typically would ride five times per week, but since the accident, he was unable to ride because any exercise increased his symptoms, as would stress, thinking, and working on the computer.

James' initial examination lasted about two hours. It consisted of a full neurological evaluation, including balance testing, eye tracking evaluations, cognitive testing, and assessments of his organ systems. Evaluating the organs provides important information about the vagus nerve and other brain regions that are associated with emotional processing and cognition.

James presented with nystagmus that was not present when seated, but appeared when he was lying down in different positions and would change depending on what position he was in. Many people are familiar with positional nystagmus that is caused by crystals that should be in one part of the inner ear, the otoliths, which then break free and move to the canals. This is a peripheral vertigo called benign positional paroxysmal vertigo (BPPV).

BPPV is associated with vertigo that lasts 30 seconds to two minutes. The treatment is a simple canal repositioning maneuver. James' nystagmus was quite different as it was from a miscalibration within the central nervous system. His challenge was unique in that it was positionally dependent and, therefore, required more advanced treatments.

The Vestibular System

The vestibular apparatus is located inside your inner ear, and it contains nerves that sense different types of movement — from bouncing on a trampoline to spinning in circles — but it is only one part of the vestibular system. The system as a whole compares information from your inner ear to information from your eyes and your body. Each of these sensory systems must work together to help create a coherent picture of who you are and where you are located in space. If this information is not working synergistically, you get what we call sensory mismatches. These sensory conflicts can lead to the following symptoms: dizziness, vertigo, nausea, motion sensitivity, visual impairment, headaches, neck pain or poor coordination and balance.

It is said that the information from the vestibular system is pervasive throughout the entire neuroaxis, which means that it has the potential to affect all functions of the body, but some areas of the brain are more intimately related to the vestibular system than others. For instance, the vestibular nuclei are located in the lower brain stem. They are right next to the vagus nerve and nausea centers. This helps explain why sometimes when we are dizzy, we get nauseous or our stomach feels funny. It is common for people who have suffered from vestibular concussions to have vertigo associated with nausea and digestive issues.

These nerve centers are also intimately related to the midline cerebellum. In the seminal book *The Cerebellum and Cognition*, Dr. Jeremy D. Schmahmann labels the midline cerebellum as a region that is strongly associated with fear and anxiety. It is also known to be intimately connected with the vestibular neurons and the vestibular system. This helps to explain why if people get anxious, they get sick to their stomach or why if someone feels ill, they feel lightheaded and dizzy.

Concussion Symptoms and Brain Regions

It is well understood that concussions can affect some areas of the brain more than others, and depending on what areas are injured, symptoms can vary from person to person.

If someone injures the frontal lobe, it is common to have more foggy thinking and challenges with decision-making. The parietal lobe is known to be associated with spatial awareness, so it makes sense that when people injure the parietal lobe, they end up feeling disoriented and out of sorts. If they injure the occipital lobe, they will frequently get problems with visual processing. The temporal lobe and insula are more associated with memory, emotion, and hallucinations.

Hallucinations are often thought to be things like hearing or seeing things that don't exist, but they are usually not that severe. There are all different types of hallucinations. For example, some people will smell things burning or will taste metal. It is more common to have these subtle hallucinations when experiencing a concussion affecting the temporal lobe. Most people do not realize that what they are sensing is coming from the concussion.

James' problems were related to his lower brainstem, and this was causing him to have symptoms associated with different positions. If we had not tested him in those different positions, it was possible to miss what was actually happening to him.

James also had two other problems that significantly affected his condition: an inability to attenuate his vestibulo-ocular reflex (VOR) and an increased cervical-ocular reflex (COR).

The VOR is a reflex very often affected by concussions. The purpose of this reflex is to stabilize your focus on a target during head movement. You can try focusing your eyes on this book and moving your head to either side. If your VOR works properly, your eyes will stay on the target while your head moves. Another way to test for VOR is to rotate in a desk chair. When you rotate to the left, your eyes should slowly drift to the right, then move quickly back to the left. Equally important, if you visually fixate on a target as the desk chair rotates, you should be able to inhibit the movement of your eyes. The inability to inhibit the VOR was a contributing factor to James' vertigo, headaches, and neck pain.

The COR reflex works very closely with the VOR. The COR is an important neurodevelopmental reflex in infants. It stabilizes their eyes in response to trunk-to-head movements. This helps them with visual targeting, but as they get older and the brain develops more, this reflex is inhibited. James' concussion injured the areas of his brain that inhibited this reflex, which caused it to become active again. This made it very difficult for him to coordinate his eye movements with his neck. His neck would get unusually tight, and his eyes would not track correctly. Before coming to our clinic, James got numerous treatments for his neck, but he could not get it to relax. His chiropractor recognized that he was not responding normally to treatments and sent him to our office for an examination. This finding was an integral part of his rehabilitation.

James' Successful Treatment Plan

James' treatment plan consisted of 30-minute treatments two times a week for six weeks. Our plan was focused mainly on vestibular rehabilitation, and we began by addressing his positional nystagmus. These treatments consisted of gaze stability exercises in the different positions that caused his nystagmus; gaze stability exercises are known to promote neuroplastic changes that improve the vestibular system and associated symptoms. We used infrared cameras on the video nystagmography system to monitor what his eyes were doing in the different positions. Then, while we monitored the nystagmus, we applied the treatment that was needed at that moment in real-time. As the nystagmus improved, we altered the therapy to what was most appropriate. These treatments resolved his positional nystagmus and associated dizziness.

This was followed by VOR attenuation therapy. We had James look at his thumb while we rotated him at a rate and vector where he could stay focused on his thumb and inhibit his VOR. As he improved, we increased the speed and amplitude of the treatments. After three visits, James' headaches went from a constant seven out of ten on the pain scale to only occurring once in the afternoon for approximately 30 minutes.

After the improvements from the first few visits, we administered COR attenuation therapy, which is similar to VOR attenuation therapy. We held James' head in place while gently rotating his body at a speed and vector where he could inhibit his COR. Once his ability to attenuate his COR improved, we performed cervical adjustments and myofascial treatments. After ten visits, James reported that his dizziness had completely resolved, and his neck pain only occurred while performing strenuous exercise.

Once the COR and VOR systems were recalibrated, James felt better and was able to return to his normal lifestyle and athletic hobbies. He stated the pain did not rise above a one out of ten, so he was referred back to his primary chiropractor to continue his wellness care.

Conclusion

Vestibular concussions are quite common, but each person's system responds in a different way. Consider how complex the vestibular system is and the fact it is involved with every other system of the neuroaxis. It is no surprise that everyone exhibits symptoms in a slightly unique manner. This makes it problematic to try to follow a formulaic treatment for every patient.

We find it very helpful to utilize our individualized approach. By understanding the complexity of the system, we allow one finding to lead us to the next relevant exam procedure. A doctor cannot perform every exam possible, so it is important to allow the exam findings to help pick which test to perform next. By approaching the exam in a dynamic manner, we work to understand each patient's unique situation.

The treatment phase of the care plan is always associated with ongoing observations and further examination as the patient's symptoms improve. This constant treatment-observation-treatment approach allows functional neurologists to solve complex symptom presentations, such as in James' case.

Dr. Cassandra Jimenez is a board-certified chiropractic neurologist currently working as lead clinician at Georgia Chiropractic Neurology Center. She obtained her bachelor's degree in Natural Science at the University of Puerto Rico in Bayamon and her Doctorate in Chiropractic from Life University. She graduated summa cum laude and was awarded the Clinic Excellence Award while also becoming valedictorian of her class. Dr. Jimenez holds a fellowship from the American Board of Vestibular Rehabilitation and has two peer-reviewed case studies published in the journal Frontiers in Neuroscience. She works as an adjunct faculty member for Life University's Chiropractic Science department.

Chapter 12

The Heart-Brain Connection
By Dr. Perry Maynard, DC, DACNB

When we go to the doctor, we usually first see our primary care doctor. If we have stomach issues, we will be referred to a GI specialist; if we have joint pain, we may be referred to a rheumatologist; and if there is a concern of heart issues, the doctor will send us to a cardiologist.

Part of what has enabled the advancements of Western medicine has been the development of specialization within healthcare. Specialization will enable doctors to spend their entire careers focused on a singular body system and allow them to master their specialty. I believe specialization brings many benefits to patients and doctors, but sometimes, we become too myopic in our studies as a healthcare system. We forget that the body is not a singular system but an entire system that is all intrinsically built off one another.

Examples of these connections become more apparent every day in discussions about the brain-gut connection or the connection between metabolic health and things like heart health and brain health. This chapter aims to shed light on the massively important link between the brain and the cardiovascular system and the autonomic nervous system (ANS), which one might call neurocardiology: the study of how the brain and heart work together and how when things go wrong in the nervous system, they can manifest in cardiovascular symptoms.

The Heart

The heart is an amazing organ of the body and is vital for life. Each day, it pumps up to 2,000 gallons of blood to oxygenate your body's cells. It receives unoxygenated blood from the body and sends it to your lungs to be oxygenated, and then back to the heart for distribution to your body. The oxygenated blood travels through the body in arteries until they reach specific tissues. The vasculature system is an intricate system of tubing that flows to every body part. To send blood through the body, we must maintain certain blood pressure. Blood pressure is supported via a few mechanisms, including contractions of the arteries or increased blood volume.

The Autonomic Nervous System

These systems are all, thankfully, automated and controlled by our ANS, which controls the cardiovascular system by sending impulses from the central nervous system (CNS) to organs within the body. Its effects on the heart include control of heart rate, control of the force of heart contraction and constriction, and dilatation of blood vessels.

Efferent and Afferent Nerves

Within the nervous system, there are efferent and afferent nerves. Efferent nerves send signals from the CNS to the effector organ, usually classified as motor signals. You also have afferent nerve fibers that take information from the periphery and bring it back to the CNS; these are classified as sensory nerves, transmitting sensory information from the body to the brain.

These same nerves are present in the ANS. Afferent, or sensory, nerves feed the brain information about blood pressure, oxygen and carbon dioxide concentration, body temperature, etc. This information is then transmitted to certain processing areas within the brain. The brain then interprets the signal and decides what type of efferent or motor signal it needs to send back into the body. The brain then decides whether to increase or decrease the heart rate depending on what is occurring.

SA and AV Nodes

The ANS can be divided into two branches: the parasympathetic and the sympathetic nervous systems. Although these systems can run independently, they are primarily modulated and regulated by the CNS. Before we get to the brain's control, let's discuss some basic cardio physiology.

There are sinoatrial nodes, SA nodes, and atrioventricular nodes, or AV nodes, in the heart. The SA node generates electrical signals to cause contraction of the atria, which is the top part of the heart, and the AV node causes contraction of the lower aspect of the heart, also known as the ventricles. These nodes work together to create electrical signals in the heart and keep a specific rhythm and rate. This is known as the heart's pacemaker — its intrinsic ability to beat and maintain a rhythm on its own.

The parasympathetic system innervates the heart via the vagus nerve, which sends signals to the AV and SA nodes, slowing the heart rate, decreasing overall cardiac output, and reducing the force of contraction of the heart. Overall, the vagus nerve appears to lower the general excitability of the heart itself.

Unlike the parasympathetic nervous system, the sympathetic nervous system affects both the heart tissue and the vascular system. It does this via specific chemical sensors, also known as alpha 1 and 2 and beta 1 and 2 adrenergic receptors. They mainly rely on epinephrine and norepinephrine to work, also known as adrenaline. These neurochemicals increase heart rate and vascular tone to increase blood pressure. Both the sympathetic and parasympathetic nervous systems are under constant control and regulation by higher-up centers in the brain.

The Medulla

The first stop for regulating ANS information is within the brainstem or, more specifically, the bottom of the brainstem — the medulla. Within your arteries, there are baroreceptors and chemoreceptors. These two sensors detect pressor changes and chemical changes occurring in the blood. This information is sent via specific sensory nerves to an area in the medulla called the nucleus tractus solitaries, or NTS. This is the first stop for information regarding the state of the cardiovascular system.

The information is then processed and fed to various other centers, including the nucleus ambiguous (NA), caudal ventral lateral medulla (CVLM), and the rostral ventrolateral medulla (RVLM). These are the parasympathetic and sympathetic outflows from the brainstem to the body. This reflex is known as the baroreceptor reflex, and its role is to maintain blood pressure throughout the body.

When we stand, gravity will pull blood into our feet, which will cause a decrease in pressure in the arteries in our neck. Decreases in pressure will change the firing rate of specific nerves back to the brain to alert it that there is a change in blood pressure. The brain then must determine if it needs to release stress chemicals to increase heart rate and blood pressure or if it needs to decrease them. When this reflex usually works, we never think twice about being able to stand up and walk around, but when one suffers a brain injury or develops an infection or autoimmune disease that negatively impacts these reflexes, then everyday life becomes exceptionally daunting.

A Higher-Up System: The Hypothalamus

You are starting to see how everything in the body has a higher-up system that controls it. This brainstem reflex we discussed is further controlled by a higher-up center called the hypothalamus.

The hypothalamus is the area of the brain concerned with maintaining homeostasis or balance within the body. It regulates body temperature and sleep-wake cycles (also known as circadian rhythms), blood sugar, thirst, and hormonal systems. It is a central part of what regulates most human bodily functions, including controlling the ANS.

It is also where things like emotional arousal can start impacting these lower-down autonomic reflexes. If you are scared, your heart rate and blood pressure may increase, or if you are embarrassed, you may get flushing of the skin. These changes occur secondary to autonomic arousal, which is happening in these higher-up brain centers. When the hypothalamus is not working optimally, you may develop sleep disturbances, hormonal issues, blood sugar problems, temperature regulation problems, and exercise intolerance.

Another Higher-Up System: The Prefrontal Cortex

So if the hypothalamus controls the brainstem autonomic systems, what regulates the hypothalamus?

That would be the cortex or, more specifically, the prefrontal cortex. The prefrontal cortex has many roles and modulates many functions throughout the CNS. This includes attention, impulse control, cognitive flexibility, working memory, and goal-directed behavior. It is one of the most developed parts of our brains and is what makes us human. The prefrontal cortex receives information from all sensory systems, creates the reality of the world around you, and decides how to interact with it. This area is very commonly affected by concussions and mild traumatic brain injuries.

What Happens When Things Go Wrong

Until there is a breakdown in the ANS, we usually don't even notice until the problems become forefront in our lives. When we stand, how many of us ever think about everything that must occur to keep gravity from taking all of our blood and pooling it in our feet, which is what happens in POTS, or postural orthostatic tachycardia syndrome? Do we ever pay attention to our body's ability to regulate body temperature with fine-tuning precision? What about simply controlling our heart rate at rest?

Unfortunately for some, these systems can break down, leading to debilitating symptoms like lightheadedness, dizziness, headaches, nausea, weakness, anxiety, diarrhea, constipation, exercise, and heat intolerance. There are various reasons these systems fail. Brain injuries, infections, autoimmune disorders, and other inflammatory issues are the most common problems that negatively affect the ANS. Brain injuries, in particular, can disrupt the pathways discussed; you have seen how tightly connected all these control centers are, so when one is disrupted, it can affect the systems under its control.

Because of the variety of symptoms that a breakdown in the ANS can cause, patients may see a variety of specialists, going from doctor to doctor but never getting to the root of the problem.

Disruption of the brain's control of the cardiovascular system can lead to the development of dysautonomia and other various symptoms. Dysautonomia is the poor regulation of the ANS, including blood pressure and heart rate. Helping individuals with dysautonomia is partially about finding what systems are feeding wrong information to the other reflexes. Once your doctor diagnoses the problem, they can plan certain treatments to try and improve the systems' function and allow them to better integrate with other systems within the brain.

As you can see, there is far more to things like heart rate and blood pressure than just our heart and arteries. Although they are essential, so is the brain in properly regulating those systems. Individuals with dysautonomia get lost in the healthcare system due to the complexity of the condition. To understand dysautonomia, one must understand the connection between the brain and the heart.

Dr. Perry Maynard is a board-certified chiropractic neurologist who specializes in the management of complex neurological cases, including post-concussive syndrome, vertigo, balance disorders, movement disorders, dysautonomia, and a variety of autoimmune conditions. Dr. Maynard has extensive education and training in concussion rehabilitation, vestibular rehabilitation, and neuroimmunology. He first became interested in neurological rehabilitation after playing Division 1 college football for Eastern Illinois University, where he experienced multiple concussions and witnessed friends and teammates suffering without answers or options for treatment. This is why he has dedicated his professional life to helping those suffering from traumatic brain injuries.

Directory

Dr. Marc Ellis, D.C. MSc, NMT, DACNB, FACFN, FABBIR
Dr. Cassandra Jimenez, DC, DACNB, FABVR
Georgia Chiropractic Neurology Center
healthybrainnow.com
Marietta, GA
770-664-4288
office@healthybrainnow.com

Dr. Kassie Kaas, DC
Valeo Health and Wellness Center
www.valeowc.com
Eden Prairie, MN
952-949-0676
drkassiekaas@gmail.com

Dr. Eric Kaplan, DC, DACNB, FACFN, FABVR, FABCDD
Kaplan Brain & Body
www.kaplandc.com
Emerson, NJ, and New York, NY
201-261-2150
info@kaplanbrainandbody.com

Dr. Lori Levy, DC, CFMP, CACCP, BA
Functional Health Unlimited
www.functionalhealthunlimited.com
Woodbury, MN
612-708-1676
drlorijokinen@gmail.com

Dr. Perry Maynard, DC, DACNB
Integrated Brain Centers
Intergratedbraincenters.com
Englewood, CO
303-781-5617
drmaynard@integratedhealthdenver.com

Dr. Mehul Parekh, DC, DACNB
Northwest Functional Neurology
www.northwestfunctionalneurology.com
Lake Oswego, OR
503-850-4526
info@northwestfunctionalneurology.com

Dr. Michael Schmidt, DC, DACNB
Missouri Functional Neurology and Chiropractic
www.mofuncneuro.com
Centralia, MO
636-486-6117
mofuncneuro@gmail.com

Dr. Clayton Shiu, PhD
The Shiu Clinic
www.shiuclinic.com
New York, NY
646-350-0165
reception.shiu@gmail.com
East Hampton, NY
631-760-7442
ehreception.shiu@gmail.com

Dr. Shane Steadman, DC, DACNB, DABCN, CNS
Integrated Brain Centers
www.integratedbraincenters.com
Englewood, CO
303-781-5617
info@integratedhealthdenver.com

Dr. Ayla Wolf, DAOM, L.Ac., Dipl O.M. (NCCAOM)
Healing Response Acupuncture & Functional Neurology
www.healingresponseneuro.com
Stillwater, MN
651-323-0005
info@healingresponseneuro.com

Amy Zellmer
Faces of TBI
www.FacesofTBI.com
The Brain Health Magazine
www.thebrainhealthmagazine.com
St. Paul, MN
amyzellmertbi@gmail.com

Meet the Collaborators

Amy Zellmer

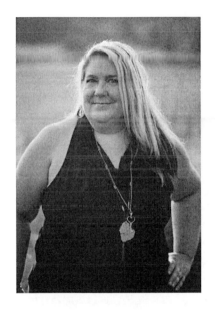

Amy is an award-winning author, speaker, and editor-in chief of *The Brain Health Magazine*, located in Minneapolis, Minnesota. Additionally, she hosts a podcast series, *Faces of TBI*, and "TBI TV" on YouTube.

Amy sustained her TBI in February of 2014 after falling on a patch of ice and landing full-force on the back of her skull. She is still recovering and understanding the full scope of her injury. She is currently working on her next book, *Creating Wellness from Within*.

Her work has frequently been featured in *Huffington Post*, *Thrive Global*, and *The Good Men Project*. She is a loud and proud advocate for TBI awareness and began the

#NOTINVISIBLE awareness campaign in 2019. She also teaches weekly brain-boosting yoga classes via Zoom.

Amy believes the healing process begins with the telling of your story and releasing everything you've been bottling up inside. Her goal is to tell other survivors' stories and share their images. TBI is an invisible disability that many don't understand. Amy wants to bring an awareness and understanding of TBI to the world and hopes people will have more compassion for those who look seemingly fine but inside are struggling with memory or cognitive issues, such as herself.

She is addicted to Starbucks, chocolate, and all things pink and glittery.

Connect with Amy:
www.facesoftbi.com
FB/TW/IG: @amyzellmer

Books by Amy Zellmer
Available on Amazon
Life with a Traumatic Brain Injury: Finding the Road Back to Normal
Embracing the Journey: Moving Forward after Brain Injury
Surviving Brain Injury: Stories of Hope and Inspiration
Concussion Discussions: A Functional Approach to Recovery after Brain Injury

Dr. R. Shane Steadman

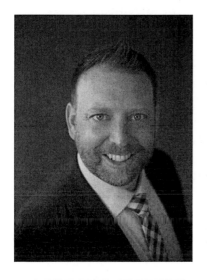

Dr. R. Shane Steadman is owner and clinic director of Integrated Brain Centers in Denver, Colorado. He is a board-certified chiropractic neurologist and a chiropractic nutritionist. He is a fellow of the American Association of Integrative Medicine. He has completed numerous hours of postgraduate and advanced studies in functional neurology and functional medicine, including functional blood chemistry, thyroid issues, neurotransmitters, and brain function, through the University of Bridgeport.

His studies also include the diagnosis and treatment of ADHD, learning disabilities, behavioral disorders, and movement disorders. He is a member of the American Chiropractic Association (ACA), the ACA Council on Neurology, the Colorado Chiropractic Association, the American Association of Integrative Medicine, the American College of Nutrition, and the International Academy of Functional Neurology and Rehabilitation.

Dr. Steadman has been lecturing since 2006, speaking to healthcare professionals on the testing and clinical applications of functional endocrinology, immunology, and blood chemistry. Dr. Steadman travels across the country lecturing on topics such as introduction to neurochemistry, applied brain concepts and clinical nutrition, autoimmune thyroid research and practice, thyroid issues, functional endocrinology, migraines, and nutritional management of neurodegenerative diseases. In 2014, Dr. Steadman was awarded Educator of the Year by the International Association of Neurology and Rehabilitation. He has also been interviewed via TV, radio, and podcast concerning various subjects on brain function. He wrote the forewords to *The Truth about Low Thyroid* by Joshua J. Redd and *Not Just Spirited* by Chynna T. Laird.

Connect with Dr. Steadman
www.integratedbraincenters.com
FB/IG @integratedbraincenters

ℛesources

Here is a small list of resources that I have compiled. I have found these sites helpful in my recovery, plus created a few of my own. I hope that they steer you in the right direction.

Brain Injury Association of America
www.biausa.org

United States Brain Injury Alliance
www.usbia.org

BrainLine
www.brainline.org

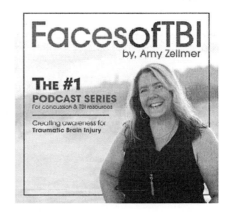

The Brain Health Magazine
www.thebrainhealthmaga-zine.com

Faces of TBI
www.facesoftbi.com

Faces of TBI Podcast Series
www.blogtalkradio.com/facesoftbi
Also available on iTunes or wherever you listen to podcasts

Facebook — Amy's TBI Tribe
www.facebook.com/groups/792052120888627

Concussion Discussions Interview Series
www.concussiondiscussions.com

Brain-Boosting Yoga Classes
www.patreon.com/amyzellmer

Life With a Traumatic Brain Injury: Finding the Road Back to Normal
www.facesoftbi.com/books
Also available on Amazon

Huffington Post **Articles**
www.huffingtonpost.com/author/amy-zellmer-634